THE DOCTOR
Father Figure or Plumber

THE DOCTOR

FATHER FIGURE OR PLUMBER

JAMES McCORMICK

CROOM HELM LONDON

Croom Helm Ltd, 2-10 St John's Road, London SW11

British Library Cataloguing in Publication Data

McCormick, J.
The doctor.
1. Physicians
I. Title
610 R130

ISBN 0-85664-593-1

Printed in Great Britain by
Biddles Ltd, Guildford, Surrey

CONTENTS

'One of the chief causes of poverty in science is imaginary wealth. The aim of science is not to open a door to infinite wisdom but to set a limit to infinite error . . . '

(Bertolt Brecht, *Galileo*.)

FOR MY PATIENTS

ACKNOWLEDGEMENTS

I am very grateful to the many colleagues who have materially affected my thinking. In particular my friends in the Royal College of General Practitioners and the members of my department; John Kevany who has broadened my horizons, Aengus O'Rourke and Shane Allwright, Denis Pereira Gray, Dorothy Robbie and Colin McCance have read, criticised and improved the manuscript. David Croom has provided encouragement, wise counsel and editorial help. Julian Tudor Hart drew my attention to the quotation from Bertolt Brecht.

Without the patience and help of Biddy, my wife, and of Teresa Farrell, who typed innumerable drafts, this book would never have been published.

FOREWORD

This is an emotional book. It expresses feeling, it relies on judgements. I would agree with J. Kenneth Galbraith that 'the denigration of value judgement is one of the devices by which scientific pretension maintains its misconceptions'.

It is written for all those who are concerned with health. It is not a textbook for professionals although I hope that they will read it.

It is idiosyncratic and represents the viewpoint of a general practitioner who has been tinged with social medicine and has some responsibility for teaching. Its distortions are in part the result of these perspectives.

It does not attempt to acknowledge more than a fraction of the sources upon which it draws. Some of these sources are known, some are buried deep in my subconscious.

It is self-indulgent because it stems from emotion. To prolong the apologia would be further indulgence.

1 THE ROLE OF THE DOCTOR

Medicine as a Profession

Professions are distinguished from trades by the length of training, the depth of special knowledge and by codes of behaviour. Medicine is different from most other professions not by virtue of the length of training (which is extremely long), or the depth of knowledge but by its code of behaviour and by its concern with people, rather than buildings, structures or accounts. This involvement with people is shared with priests, nurses, teachers, social workers and to some extent with lawyers. It is not characteristic of architects, actuaries, accountants and engineers.

Professional codes are fundamentally of two sorts, those that protect the profession itself and those that are held to protect the client. The first sort establishes scales of fees, controls competition and lays down educational criteria for entry. Rules are enforced by disciplinary measures vested in the profession itself. The majority of professional people, excluding nurses, most doctors in the United Kingdom and a few other special categories, are not employees: that is, they do not receive a pay packet determined in negotiation with management. Their income is maintained without the need to organise as a trade union and this, for many, is one of the distinguishing marks of professional status.

When doctors' incomes depended on fees, professional ethics were largely concerned with mechanisms which controlled competition for patients. These 'ethical' matters, better described as professional etiquette, were and are concerned with the maintenance of a profession's position of privilege and the safeguarding of its autonomy. One important way in which this is achieved is by control of admission. The emphasis upon training and the necessary qualifications, usually obtained by examination, is reasonably portrayed as protecting society from the quack and the charlatan: it also serves to protect the professions themselves.

Medicine, in common with other caring professions – with the priesthood and to some extent with teachers – inherits a further and different sort of ethical responsibility which is concerned with service, a commitment to people or pupils which transcends any written contract of duties and responsibilities. This has an ancient lineage which extends backwards in our culture to the Greek civilisation and beyond, and which is enshrined, for medicine, in the Hippocratic Oath.

The Thesis

The thesis of this book is that doctors are neglecting this second sort of ethical responsibility. As a result, they are in danger of losing a special position in society, are in danger of being rejected and are failing to make their full contribution to the well-being of their fellow men and women.

This has been due in part to the impact of the scientific revolution, which led doctors, and many others, to believe that the growth of scientific knowledge and technical expertise held the key to the solution of all human problems. This view is no longer popular but its effects are persistent, particularly in medical education.

It has been due, in part, to changes in our society, particularly the movement towards greater egalitarianism and equality of educational opportunity. This has been accompanied by a rejection of authority and a reluctance to invest any section of society with special, sacerdotal or inherited position.

Lastly, most doctors in the United Kingdom no longer determine their incomes in a free enterprise economy but are employed by the state: directly, in the case of hospital staff, indirectly in the case of general practitioners, who still cling to independent contractor status. This has forced doctors to organise as a trade union in order to pursue negotiation with management. In other countries, where doctors are not state-employed, increasing involvement of the state as the major funding source for health services has led to confrontations with the profession. The doctors' efforts to maintain their incomes, which in most of these countries are large, have been perceived by society as being in conflict with their conception of doctors as a group of people marked out by a vocation to serve.

The following chapters describe this relationship and the role doctors play in our society in somewhat greater detail. This thesis is the framework within which the portrait has been painted.

The Role of the Doctor

Although medicine has been a traditional university discipline, its scientific base is relatively young. The position of doctors in the past did not rest on their ability to influence the course of disease – they were largely unable to do so – but upon their role in society. They were perceived as possessing special knowledge, sapiential authority, and as being able to mediate between the patient and his disease. They were expected to be concerned, to put the patient's interest before their own and to be bound by a special code of behaviour which differentiated them from other men. 'Medicine was, at its best, deeply respected as a learned profession.'[1]

The scientific physician concerned primarily with diagnosis and to a lesser extent with its corollaries of treatment and cure is apt to see his role as confined within relatively narrow boundaries. As a result, he has progressively neglected the care of the aged, the chronic sick and the handicapped. His inability to cure is a reproach rather than a challenge: it is in conflict with his role; he tends to believe that he has nothing to offer. His energies and his enthusiasm are bent to the solution of problems rather than their containment.

Ill people are not just disordered machinery. If therapy always promised cure, if ageing and death were not a fact, if human beings were not dependent on others, a mechanistic approach would answer their needs. In reality they need love as much as they need therapy, particularly as so much therapy is needless or ineffective.

Throughout the western world there is evidence of a conflict between doctors and society. One way of attempting to explain or understand this conflict is to assume a difference between doctors' conception of their role and society's view of what doctors should do and how they should behave. This difference may depend upon different ideas of the nature of health, disease and illness.

Most doctors, particularly the general practitioners and hospital doctors who represent the profession to the public, view their role as the diagnosis, management, treatment and cure of disease. Reduced to its lowest common denominator this is an approach which not surprisingly relies on machinery and applied technology.

It does however ignore the essential features of the state of being ill. The onset of symptoms of dis-ease interferes with the ability to function normally and often carries with it the fear that the disorder may persist or lead to death. Illness threatens autonomy. The response to this situation varies in accordance with the severity of the symptoms, perceptions of their meaning and beliefs about the nature of disease.

The first reaction of those who are ill is withdrawal into a place of safety; an instinctive need to retreat into a private cocoon of suffering, cut off from the outside world and isolated from normal concerns. This is often accompanied or followed by a need for reassurance that all will be well, which in the first instance takes the form of seeking advice from relations or friends and the taking of some remedy – usually something which has been bought over the counter rather than prescribed. If the symptoms are very severe or if they are interpreted as heralding serious disease, professional help is invoked at an early stage. If the symptoms are mild and unthreatening, professional advice may not be needed but it still may be necessary to see a doctor in order to continue an entitlement to be regarded as sick. If the cause is obvious, a broken arm or an infected finger, there is relatively little anxiety and relatively little doubt about appropriate action and the doctor or the hospital may expect to be automatically involved.

Those who are ill may have real difficulty in viewing their illness rationally and dispassionately. They are frequently beset with fears which have no basis in reason and which have their roots in vestiges of scientific knowledge garnished with old wives' tales.

The ill require from their doctors something more than accurate diagnosis and appropriate treatment. Our doctors are not trained to provide reassurance, to comfort and to care. This is not to say that they always or even often fail to do so but means that the bulk of their training has been built around a mechanistic model and that learning to care comes by accident; by the natural tendency of the taught to model themselves on their teachers rather than as a result of deliberate intent.

'Father Figure or Plumber'

The title of this section derives from a statement made by a social worker at a meeting called to discuss the goals of medical education.[2] The statement was: 'I don't want a father figure, I want a good human plumber.' This choice has been differently expressed as the choice between engineer and priest.[3]

'I don't want a father figure' rejects the authoritarianism, the superior position of doctors relative to their patients. 'I want a good human plumber' is a plea for equality, a plea for control. It also implies that disease can usefully be equated with disordered machinery and that mechanistic solutions are applicable to the problems of those who choose to come to doctors.

My theme is that doctors are in danger of getting the worst of both worlds. Retaining an authoritative paternalism to which they seem to have forfeited the right, they also demonstrate that they are indifferent human plumbers. Unless they re-examine their role and unless they succeed in establishing a better relationship with the society which they serve, their potential and the potential of health services to improve the quality of human life will be substantially diminished.

2 THE NATURE OF HEALTH

Health

This chapter is, in a sense, a digression from the theme. It is a necessary digression because a book which is concerned with doctors cannot escape reference to health, disease, illness and sickness.

Health is a conceptual term and does not lend itself to simple definition.[1] Health can be conceived as the absence of disease. This is the concept which is favoured by the majority of doctors. From it stems a very clear and simple notion of their role as the diagnosis and treatment of disease as it affects the individual patient. It is the basis of the now much denigrated medical model which conceives disease and its management in mechanistic terms. The major, some would maintain almost the sole, thrust of medical education is tied to this concept. Medical students spend almost all their undergraduate careers studying the structure and function of the human body, its disorders and their therapy. Because this concept of health focuses on the individual it tends to neglect collective health. Because of its emphasis on the management of established disease it neglects prevention. Because it views disease in mechanistic terms it ignores the fact that human beings are sentient organisms existing in a social environment: it denies wholism. In its aspirations it denies the inevitability of death and the relentless processes of ageing. Nonetheless it has been the basis for the advancement of medical science and it is a concept shared to some extent by many others besides doctors, particularly those who seek good human plumbers.

For many people health is negatively conceived as the

absence of symptoms of disease. Few can conjure up enthusiasm for the often quoted definition of the World Health Organisation, 'health is a state of complete physical, mental and social well-being, not merely the absence of disease or infirmity'. The springtime euphoria of such a state of positive health seems to bear little relationship to the nature of our journey from the cradle to the grave.

For a few, and for a small group of undervalued doctors working in social medicine and the public health service, health is a matter of environmental control. It is argued, with good reason, that the environment – using the word in its widest sense – is the major determinant of health. Health depends upon having enough (of the right sort) to eat; protection from infectious disease by immunisation and proper hygiene; protection from accidents by legislation; the provision of clean air and water, and the early diagnosis of presymptomatic disease in 'healthy' populations. Health depends upon a job, a house, and being loved.

It is generally accepted that health services have a duty to care as well as cure. This is usually thought of in terms of long-continued care. The care of the handicapped and the elderly rather than the care of the acutely ill. In a sense care is conceived of as the residual duty when cure or restoration of health has been admitted as impossible.

An increasingly popular concept of health sees health as functional capacity, as adaptation of disability rather than its eradication.[2] Quite apart from the necessity of living with the results of accidents or with the continuing discomfort of some chronic diseases, all of us have to come to terms with ageing. While it is true that medicine and more particularly surgery can alleviate and sometimes eliminate discomfort and disability, success is in many instances partial. Under these circumstances successful living may depend upon a refusal to agree to surrender the individual autonomy that is implicit in choosing to be sick. This is the spirit which is universally admired in those who surmount their handicaps.

Successful living depends upon the ability to adapt to change: for many it is necessary to adapt to different climates and different cultures. All of us have to cope with bereavement and ultimately with death. Health is the ability to live autonomously: health is successful coping.

It is clear that this is my preferred definition and that this must in turn influence my view of the doctor's role in the promotion and maintenance of health. This definition carries the implication that health is an expression of an individual's ability to survive rather than a state that is in the gift of either doctors or a beneficent government.

Disease, Illness and Sickness

Disease can be much more readily defined. There are, nonetheless, two different and distinct approaches. The first concentrates on the dis-ease aspects. This has the advantage of admitting a wide variety of maladaptations to the category of disease states. By concentrating on the symptomatic aspects it ignores the fact that quite advanced changes can remain symptomless. The alternative is to regard disease as the presence of identifiable abnormality rather than the existence of symptoms and this is the sense in which I will use the term confining the word illness to the subjective perception of dis-ease.

The problem with this definition is that it depends upon being able to determine normality. Biological characteristics tend to be distributed equally above and below an average value. For example, most adult men are about five feet nine inches in height: those who are very tall or very short may have had some disorder of growth or may be extreme examples of the 'normal' distribution.

Disease usually includes the degenerative changes which accompany ageing, the reference point for normality being young adults. Almost all people over eighty have lens degenerations, cataracts, which are usual or 'normal' in a population of eighty-year-olds but very unusual and clearly abnormal in young adults.

High 'normal' levels of both blood cholesterol and blood pressure are associated with an increased risk of coronary heart disease, and in the case of blood pressure of stroke. There is as a result a temptation to lower levels of blood cholesterol and blood pressure which are biologically normal. Similarly the overweight, whose life expectancy is reduced, may be urged to diet and exercise more.

Mental disease poses special problems because most of what is categorised as mental disease is not associated with demonstrable physical abnormality. The diagnosis usually rests on symptoms or on disordered behaviour. Clearly, judgements about the significance of symptoms or the abnormality of behaviour are subjective and depend upon the perceptions and cultural background of the doctor rather than on measurable absolutes. Behaviour that is normal in Samoa may be deviant in Tooting.

Illness is the presence of symptoms, the subjective experience of dis-ease. Many diseases, including such important conditions as cancers, anaemias and diabetes, may be symptomless for long periods of time. Illness may be present in the absence of physical disease. Unhappiness, anxiety, tiredness, loss of libido are symptoms often brought to doctors. They are seldom associated with any physical abnormality.

Sickness on the other hand is not simply the presence of dis-ease, it is a role sanctioned by society. Those who choose to become sick are exempted from normal social responsibilities. In return for this exemption they are expected to behave as sick people, to seek to become well (it is assumed that they cannot become well by an act of will) and they must co-operate in treatment usually prescribed by doctors.[3]

It is not permissible to say 'I will not go to work, go to school, wash the dishes.' It is entirely acceptable to plead that 'I am sick and therefore I cannot.' All of us have had the experience of a minor illness which has allowed us to retire to the comfort and security of a warm bed. On awaking from a refreshing sleep we have been faced with Bovril and a cream cracker when we would have happily demolished dinner. Having dinner is conditional on taking a share of the washing-up.

Many of those who are ill may refuse to become sick. Similarly sickness may be prolonged because of its advantages although illness may have ceased and although the individual was never diseased.

3 THE DOCTOR AND THE PATIENT

Introduction

In the middle of the last century, most people lived and died without the help or hindrance of doctors. Doctors worked mainly in the cities and made their living by attending the middle class. Victorian philanthropy was in full flood, hospitals and other institutions to care for the sick and deserving poor were being founded daily, each adorned with a prestigious board of governors. A glance at a popular Dublin directory, published in 1838, lists in addition to hospitals, societies and organisations as various as the Asylum for Aged Printers, the Society for Superseding The Necessity of Climbing Boys in Sweeping Chimneys, the Charitable Society for the Relief of Sick and Indigent Roomkeepers of All Religious Persuasions, and Simpson's Hospital, for the Reception of Poor, Decayed, Blind and Gouty Men.

The primary function of hospitals, originally hospices, was care; care of the deserving and sick poor. Nobody thought of a hospital as a place to be cured, it was a place to die or if one was fortunate, to survive. The middle class and the well-to-do would not have dreamt of going into hospital. Doctors, as part of the philanthropy of the age, gave their services for nothing. They were however able to enlarge their experience and to teach their students. The tradition that consultants provided a service to teaching hospitals as 'honoraries' while making their living from private practice persisted until the institution of the National Health Service in 1948.

The age of scientific medicine, beginning with Harvey in the seventeenth century, gradually gained momentum in the latter half of the last century. Simpson began to use chloroform, Lister pioneered antisepsis and Pasteur's fundamental researches into the nature of micro-organisms paved the way for a true understanding of the nature of infection. As the momentum increased and as each new year saw new discoveries – insulin, liver for the treatment of pernicious anaemia, sulphonamides, penicillin, the expectations of both doctors and society of scientific medicine became more and more unrealistic. The optimism of the Victorian age, despite two world wars, has persisted in respect of science, technology and medicine. It is by no means dead but there has been, especially in the last ten years, a powerful counter-current of disillusion.

It has been said of medical knowledge that it has a half-life of five years; within five years half of the present body of knowledge will have been discarded or substantially modified. Yet the growth of knowledge has not been accompanied by a dramatic improvement in health. The impact of new knowledge grows progressively less. Implicit in conception is death, and medicine cannot aspire to do more than 'help us to come safely into the world and to leave it comfortably'.[1] One of the reasons that society is disillusioned with its doctors is their failure to meet unrealistic expectations.

Even more important than failure to meet unreal expectations has been failure to meet those that are normal or traditional. In all societies the professional healer, witch doctor, shaman, or general practitioner has been accorded high status. This was in recognition, in part, of the possession of special knowledge and skills but it also recognised a priestly role, a sacerdotal authority which was both mysterious and mystical. Doctors were not as other men and were expected not only to possess knowledge but also to subscribe to a special and demanding code of behaviour.

The first demand which is made of doctors is that they should put the patient first. They are expected to subjugate their personal life to the needs of their patients. It is assumed that surgeons will complete operations with both care and concentration regardless of competing private commitments. Because doctors can sometimes save life they should be prepared to respond promptly to emergencies. If somebody is dying, is in danger of death or has suffered an accident, being off duty, in bed or busy in the garden provides no adequate excuse for not responding to the call for help. If doctors are not prepared to get out of bed, they should forfeit their special position.

A privileged position is also conditional on a high standard of personal behaviour. This is enshrined in legislation which empowers the General Medical Council to remove doctors' names from the Register, and thereby deny them the right to practise. A high standard of personal behaviour is more than successful evasion of criminal prosecution or of being brought before the disciplinary committee of the General Medical Council.

Doctors are not expected to be dirty, foul-mouthed or rude. They should not get drunk, except as medical students. They should not cheat or fornicate. They should not display cupidity. If all these conditions are satisfied, doctors are likely to be guaranteed high status and the income that goes with it.

In the light of what has been said it is not surprising that the major criticisms of the profession have been about behaviour rather than about technical competence. Complaints within the NHS are about failures to visit, about rudeness, about thoughtlessness, not about technical competence.[2] Deputising services and rigid appointment systems have aroused wrath. Strike action, either real or threatened, has been seen as non-professional conduct.

Medical Education

Medical schools, by emphasising with good reason the scientific aspects of practice, have unwittingly diminished concern for patients as people. The strength of academic departments in clinical subjects has been the rigorous application of scientific method to the diagnosis and management of disease. This encouraged a mechanistic approach and tended to undervalue 'soft' areas, aspects that are not easily measured. Until very recently neither teachers nor taught had any knowledge of behavioural science or sociology and psychiatry had only begun to emerge as a major subject. It sometimes seemed as if patients had ceased to exist as people. Jenny Smith, housewife of middle age, happily married, who has problems with her daughter and her mother, is still good looking, terrified of cancer and frightened of surgery, is transmuted into the breast biopsy in bed four.

Medical students' attitudes change during the course of their studies. One investigator

> tried, over a few years, to evaluate the 'image of the physician' as seen by students prior to their admission in the medical school: in their fourth year of study; in their sixth year; and, finally, as young physicians. It became clear through this study that candidates applying to the medical school are motivated primarily by their wish to become doctors caring for patients, to function, after termination of their study period, as healers in the traditional sense of the word. During the six-year period of study a gradual change in their attitudes and motivation occurs, leading, at the end, to a change in their basic outlook. They become less motivated to function as healers, develop to some degree even a cynical attitude in this respect, and begin to think in respect of their future in terms of scientists and researchers, who appear to them to be of a higher status in society – and especially in the society of the medical school, in the university establishments, and in the appreciation of their own colleagues. . . . It is quite clear that the student's change of his own future image as a physician is determined by the example of his teachers and by the framework in which his clinical training is carried out.[3]

Control

In general practice, even when payment is not by fee, the contract between patient and doctor is a personal one. In hospital, especially in the case of non-fee-paying patients, the contract is to an extent with the institution rather than with the individual surgeon or physician. While clinical responsibility ultimately rests with the consultant, he or she may not perform the operation and may never see the patient. The members of the team, registrars, house-officers, interns and medical students are answerable, not to the patient, but to the consultant. Nurses are answerable to ward-sisters and nursing officers, domestic staff to the domestic supervisor. Happiness, promotion and income are not dependent upon the regard of patients but upon the approbation of peers and superiors. Patient comfort may be sacrificed to sister's insistence on a tidy ward before consultant or matron make their rounds. A houseman, fearing the wrath of his chief if a certain investigation has not been completed, is unlikely to omit it even if the patient objects.[4]

The loss of patients' ability to control their doctors has diminished the responsiveness of the profession. Doctors are trained in an environment where they are encouraged by example and precept to develop high standards of scientific and technical competence. Their qualification and subsequent promotion depends upon demonstrating to their superiors their knowledge and skills. As a result they are in danger of perceiving their role as primarily technical and of rejecting the many other demands that we would make of our doctors.

Patients are at a great disadvantage in trying to control their doctors. A majority, though possibly a diminishing number, of doctors are recruited from the higher social classes and their values and behaviours are largely those of the upper middle class. In the USA, where income is more closely linked with status, doctors are equally clearly differentiated from the majority of their potential patients. In the United Kingdom, particularly in the country, older people conscious of the niceties of social hierarchy will accord to the doctor a considerable measure of respect, only marginally less than that paid to the squire. People may still use 'Sir' in their speech, and within Roman Catholic communities, doctors have the experience of being inadvertently addressed as 'Father'.

Those disadvantaged in terms of status and social class still feel the need to behave in ways that will be approved by their doctors, because lacking that approval their prospect of gaining their objectives is substantially diminished. This need to be approved extends beyond behaviour to matters of dress, and personal cleanliness. Occasionally, when I have sought to examine a patient I have been told, 'I am sorry doctor but I didn't come prepared for an examination.' Bedrooms are still cleaned in anticipation of the doctor's arrival, and in emergencies, concern about the state of the house sometimes seems to be greater than concern about the state of the patient.

This need, to be thought well of by the doctor, is not confined to those whose status or class is different and it stems, in part at least, from the supplicant posture. Doctors express it very strongly in their own illnesses: their greatest fear in seeking advice from colleagues about themselves is that they should be regarded as nuisances, hypochondriacal, neurotic or not respectably and really diseased. This in part explains their reluctance to seek help, particularly in the case of psychiatric disorder, but they may also deny other serious symptoms such as those of coronary heart disease.[5]

With the sole exception of the disappearing home visit, doctor/patient transactions take place on the doctor's territory. It was Keith Hodgkin who first made me aware that for man, as well as for robins, territory was important.[6] His sage advice, as I recollect it, was 'If you must be rude to people, don't be rude to them in their own homes'. Some general practitioners, aware of the effect of white coats and stainless steel, have concentrated on giving their surgeries or offices a domestic atmosphere and have tried to keep the more impressive and threatening pieces of equipment out of sight. Few hospitals attempt this, and like most health centres, at best produce a bright, chintzy but nonetheless clinical atmosphere. The mahogany, leather, antique oils or good prints of the Harley Street consulting room are in remarkable contrast to the bare benches of some out-patient departments.

Once admitted to hospital disadvantages multiply. The patient is stripped of personal identity by being unclothed. Both pyjamas and nightdress offer only limited possibilities of maintaining identity. The bedside locker, the total extent of individual territory, can be used to signal the degree to which one is loved in the outside world. The expensive carnations, the array of get-well cards, the peaches and the casually placed *War and Peace* are all important and demonstrate that if 'I am nobody in here, I am certainly somebody outside.'

There are other disadvantages of being in bed and not the least is horizontal posture. Nobody who is lying down can control a transaction with somebody who is standing up. The temptation, denied the ability to stand up, is to turn away and agree to submit to whatever ensues.

Few hospital wards make any concessions to privacy other than curtains. Neither curtains, nor moveable screens, in any way provide protection against noise or allow the possibility of private conversation. Even in a single room it may be difficult to talk to the consultant if he is accompanied by his juniors, the ward sister and the social worker. Recently, a patient confessed to me: 'No, I did not tell the doctor. Sister was looking at me in such a funny way.'

A doctor writing in the *Lancet* about his personal experience of being in hospital begins: 'I would say that what demoralises the patient in the first place is the loss of personal identity.'[7] He goes on:

> patients inevitably have the feeling that they have not only lost freedom in the broad sense of the term, but that they have also been deprived of the right to take decisions. . . . I believe that the loss of decision-making is probably the heaviest blow of all to most patients' morale. I was fortunate to be in a side-ward where I was, in fact, able to take some decisions which may seem laughably trivial now, but at the time were to me, in my confined world, matters of the greatest importance. It happened to be in the heatwave last summer, and I was able to decide for myself how much window I would have open by day and again by night; before setting the window for the night, I consulted the thermometer. Thus I already had two decisions to make daily, and there was also the degree to which the door should be open, an apparently even more trivial matter but one which assumed very satisfactory importance, since it was left entirely for me to decide.

In both the UK and the USA medical education concentrates on the diagnosis, investigation and treatment of physical disease. Psychiatry is acknowledged as being important. General practice has some place in most schools. Nevertheless most doctors, including general practitioners, have an image of their role which was elegantly described as follows: 'To obtain his greatest satisfaction the doctor usually wants to find a patient with a serious, acute illness that has interesting features – elicited and recognised by him with great acumen – and one who responds rapidly, completely and gratefully to proper therapy.'[8]

Further evidence on this score has recently been published by G.V. Stimson.[9] He asked several hundred general practitioners, mostly under 35, to give a brief sketch of those patients who cause the least trouble and those who cause the most trouble. The profile that emerged was as follows:

LEAST TROUBLE	MOST TROUBLE
Illness	
healthy	feel ill
specific symptoms	vague symptoms
organic/physical	psychological/psychiatric
easy to diagnose	hard to diagnose
can be treated	social problem
easy to manage	hard to manage
get better	do not get better
Patient Behaviour	
do not consult	consult
can judge when to consult	cannot judge when to consult
undemanding	demanding
do not take time	take up time
clearly present problems	vaguely present problems
have confidence in doctor	do not trust doctor
accept limits to doctor's skill	do not accept limits to skill
grateful	ungrateful
want to get better/accept illness	do not want to get better/deny illness
accept judgement of doctor	critical of doctor
follow advice	do not follow advice
co-operative	un-co-operative

Social Competence	
intelligent	low IQ
with common sense	lack common sense
can cope	'acopic'
happy	unhappy
settled	unsettled, lonely, insecure
local	from elsewhere
adequate	inadequate
busy/working	idle/malingerer
good homes and circumstances	poor social circumstances

These lists confirm that doctors are unhappy if their authority is challenged or if they are unable to see themselves as therapeutically active and effective. It is also clear that socio-economic deprivation and things that are associated with it tend to categorise patients as troublesome or 'bad'. There are other categories of 'bad' patients. Academics are 'bad'. Doctors find dons difficult because of their insistence on questioning in detail the benefits, dangers and possible ill effects of investigation or treatment. They refuse to recognise the doctor as the fountainhead of wisdom and generally wish to examine the evidence for themselves and having done so to make autonomous and, sometimes, what appear to doctors to be stupid decisions.[10]

There is a good deal of evidence, all consistent, which shows that the higher social classes make better use of and have effectively readier access to services within the NHS. Doctors also spend more time with those of higher social class.[11] On the other hand, the single homeless in our cities who qualify as troublesome under almost all heads, except those of consulting frequently and being female, fail to use any services at all.

As general practice becomes more highly organised, the underprivileged or troublesome patient has to deal not only with doctors but with receptionists, secretaries, nurses, health visitors and social workers. If the doctor labels a patient as troublesome or 'bad', it is certain that at the very least the reception staff, in order to protect the doctor, will also attach that label and try to discourage or reject the patient's efforts to see him. This happens insidiously. The doctor may, on being told that Mrs Smith has arrived without an appointment, respond by saying 'Oh! Not again!' This may, in fact, be a complaint about the doctor's lot rather than either a criticism of the receptionist or a rejection of Mrs Smith.

One of the mechanisms frequently adopted to deal with 'troublesome' patients is to refer them to other agencies, especially social workers. This act of rejection, multiplied many times, results in patients, usually by this time stigmatised as inadequate, bouncing from agency to agency and never achieving any help towards a useful solution.

Hospital staff also categorise patients as 'good' and 'bad'. The worst patients are those who seek to discharge themselves against advice. This not only challenges the wisdom and authority of the staff but is ungrateful 'after all that we have done'. Most, if not all, of Stimson's characteristics of troublesome patients are also valid in hospital. Physical disease is 'good', mental disease is 'bad'; drug addicts are 'bad', lung cancer is 'good'. This last example is interesting in that a drug addiction caused by injudicious prescribing by doctors is 'bad', whereas lung cancer caused by addiction to cigarettes is 'good'.

In brief, patients are at a disadvantage in attempting to influence the way in which doctors behave towards them or in ensuring that doctors respond to their needs. Most doctor/patient relationships bear more similarity to that between parent and child than to that between equal adults. Nonetheless patients have methods of influencing their doctors, just as children have means of getting their way.

The Patient's Choice

The need for control depends upon the nature of the illness. When the illness is severe, life-threatening or requires emergency surgery, there are no problems in abrogating autonomy and consenting to complete dependence. The less certain the benefits of treatment the more important autonomy becomes.

The mechanisms by which patients can exert a measure of control are limited. The most obvious is by exercising choice. In the past a successful doctor was a doctor with a large practice, a doctor whom many patients chose. Some of these doctors were denigrated by their peers as fashionable, which implied that their skills had more to do with a successful doctor/patient relationship, than professional competence.

The exercise of choice only becomes an effective method of control if changing doctors or not choosing a particular individual hurts: it must hurt either the doctor's pride or his pocket. When I began practice in Ireland, I had two patients. I arranged for them to arrive simultaneously in order that I would be seen to be busy. My objectives when seeing them were as much to satisfy their hopes, to persuade them of my concern and my competence, as to cure their illness. If they left me dissatisfied and disappointed, there was little likelihood that they would persuade their friends and relations to transfer their allegiance to me. As I was paid a fee for each item of service, the loss of a neurotic, hypochondriacal or chronically ill patient substantially diminished my income. These realities prompted a response to demands even when they might be thought unreasonable. A consequence of an investment in wooing patients is a feeling of substantial hurt when a colleague's car is seen outside a prized patient's door. As time passes, the knowledge grows that patients do and should change doctors, but it requires great maturity to view the desertion of a patient with undisturbed equanimity. One of the advantages of beginning practice in a competitive situation is that the importance of satisfying patients is learned early and behaviours that develop in response to this need are likely to persist for a lifetime.

In the NHS general practitioners are paid by means of a capitation fee, a sum of money paid annually in respect of each individual on the doctor's list. The capitation payable for the elderly is larger in recognition of their higher demand for services. In addition various fixed sums are payable as practice allowances and seniority payments. Special fees may be claimed for night work, family planning and insurance examinations. A doctor may hold appointments as police surgeon, clinical assistant within hospital or factory doctor. In these circumstances the loss of a single patient or even a family has little impact on income. If the family which decides to change generates a high demand for services, especially domiciliary visits, their loss may represent a net financial gain.

Private patients who decide to change do not have to inform the doctor of their decision and as a result seldom do so. In the NHS, bureaucracy, for good reasons, makes it necessary for the patients to inform the doctor of their decision. Generally speaking, people are reluctant to change their doctor. This reluctance can be explained in a variety of ways. In part it is fear of the unknown – the devil that you know is better than the devil you don't. A change involves discarding a relationship which, while it may have turned sour, still exists. Sometimes it is felt that the doctor's wrath at being deserted will follow them and haunt their relationship with their new doctor. This is not entirely fantasy as in every area there are a few families labelled as 'bad' or undesirable, whom no doctor will accept. These unfortunates are allocated to practitioners and provide evidence of an effective collusion between doctors to stigmatise some of their patients.

The decision to change doctors implies the possibility of real choice. In small communities, served mainly by a single partnership or group, choice may be limited to deciding which partner to see, but even this discretion may be reduced by rigid appointment systems or the efforts of the seniors to divert work to junior partners, trainees or assistants. In the NHS, unless list size diminishes appreciably, the less work a doctor does the less his expenses and the more his free time. The transfer of a patient to a partner or junior is a net gain unless his workload becomes so small that his partners complain. The loss of a patient can still wound a doctor's pride but rationalisations which effectively soothe are readily available.

Not only may patients be denied choice of practitioner they may also be denied choice of consultant. There are several reasons for this. Patients are usually, but by no means inevitably, less well informed about the relative strengths and weaknesses of specialists and will seek the guidance of their general practitioner. A consultant who wishes to build up his private practice wisely concentrates on wooing the doctors: if the doctor receives a good service he will refer patients. If he receives tardy reports or is treated in an offhand manner, rather than as an equal colleague, he is unlikely to choose that specialist again.

In an age of increasing specialisation choice is inevitably limited. There are, in any one local hospital, unlikely to be more than one or two doctors whose special skills are appropriate to a particular problem. Real choice only exists if the patient is prepared to go to London, or some other major centre, as a private patient. As a result a few specialists can, despite inconsiderate behaviour, continue to have many patients referred to them.

Fees

The direct payment of a fee improves the patient's ability to control the transaction. The survival of private practice is not only due to the desire to purchase privacy in hospital. It survives because it is recognised that the payment of a fee creates a contract between doctor and patient and that in some degree value for money is assured. Few people believe that they purchase a different order of competence but they know that they buy greater consideration, the right to ask questions and to demand answers. Fee paying does not produce equality but it improves the patient's position. Until recently, doctors worked fairly hard to maintain the myth that fees were unimportant and that the intrusion of money into the consultation was, at the least, vulgar. Many patients visiting Harley Street were simultaneously afraid of what it might cost and afraid to raise the sordid topic. Accounts, sometimes very tardily sent, were the rule. If payment was made at the time, this was negotiated with the secretary not with the doctor himself. Many of my patients who saw specialists privately were very reticent about enquiring what it would cost and did not see their relationship with the doctor, whom they were employing, as being similar to that which they might have with their plumber. No only did they not seek estimates for the work to be done, but they were slow to complain and reluctant to change doctors. Changing doctors was not all as easy as sacking plumbers, and the decision, or even the thought of change, was seen as conflicting with medical ethics. It was difficult to persuade patients that as they were employing doctors and paying them fees they had the right to seek estimates of cost, ask for information and to change doctors if they were dissatisfied. I remember one woman who said to me, 'You must be surprised that I have never invited you or your wife to my house.' When I demurred she went on to explain that their family doctor had been their friend and that when her mother had been ill, this friendship had prevented them insisting upon a second opinion when they felt it necessary. She regarded her mother's death as being an unnecessary consequence of the special relationship with their doctor and had decided that in future her relationship with her doctor would be confined to a professional contract.

Doctors more often nowadays seek payment in cash. While this is explained as the result of the high cost of administering and posting accounts, it is perceived and resented by those whose wages are subject to PAYE as at least creating the opportunity for tax evasion. Sometimes a doctor, especially a consultant, may effectively find his status reduced by being offered immediate payment in cash. 'I know you would prefer cash' accompanied by a wink leaves the unfortunate physician with no option other than to accept or to launch into a pompous and ludicrous account of his honesty.

The very rich use money to command doctors and are generally successful, there being a tacit agreement that if the doctor responds to their beck and call, bills, even large ones, will be paid. As they remain firmly in control and take the decisions, they may purchase, at considerable cost, a particularly bad form of medicine.

The very few people in society who perceive their status as higher than that of doctors, freed from the inhibitions that affect others, often successfully control their doctors, even without recourse to paying a fee. This is true in lesser degree throughout the social spectrum and the middle class have been shown to make more effective use of doctors than social classes 4 and 5. As a young man I was advised that the secret of success as a doctor was to 'treat your duchesses as charladies and your charladies as duchesses': it remains good advice.

A successful method of obtaining some control which is often used, particularly in more rural areas, is the giving of presents. Presents, once received, alter the relationship and are an effective bribe. Offered as tokens of gratitude, eggs, socks, a bottle of whisky or a turkey make it very difficult for the doctor to refuse requests for attention. It is almost impossible to refuse a gift offered in gratitude, sometimes at considerable sacrifice. In general, doctors accept both the gifts and the consequences with good grace. This cynical view overstates the case: it would be wrong to impute base motives to all those who show their gratitude by giving. Gifts are often a recognition of what is perceived as unusual, exceptional, or sometimes in the case of legacies, continued concern.

Litigation

The threat of litigation is an unhappy method of seeking control. In these islands litigation is still uncommon and when a good case exists it is usually settled out of court. Malpractice insurance remains cheap. In the USA extremely costly litigation is common and insurance is either unobtainable or hideously expensive. This state of affairs is reflected in doctors' fees which are pushed still higher. Most seriously it distorts medical practice. Doctors preoccupied with guarding against a law suit are obliged to undertake investigations which are expensive and occasionally unpleasant and which make little or no contribution to the good management of disease. Decisions as to what constitute neglect or malpractice tend to be made in the light of the evidence of expert witnesses. Sometimes expert witnesses disagree: sometimes the perspectives of the expert which usually derive from a highly specialised standpoint, hence their expert status, are not really relevant. What is good practice for nephrologists, who deal exclusively with cases referred to them, may be bad practice for family doctors.

An American lawyer talking to doctors, some of whom he had defended in malpractice suits, went to the heart of the problem when he said:

> Let's start with the most obvious – your relationship (or lack of one) with your patient. Isn't it strange that the person who first comes to you in complete confidence, fully prepared to refer to you fondly as "my doctor" is

> the very same person who sues the heck out of you.
>
> Quite obviously, somewhere along the line, something went wrong to cause such a wonderful start in a mutually beneficial relationship to end up fraught with suspicion, frustration and anger.

He continues, 'You can blame anyone or anything you want – the law, lawyers, courts, juries, insurance companies, or the changing times. But if you don't examine yourself, your patient and how the two of you are doing in your human relationship, you will be putting the blame in the wrong place.'[12]

Perhaps doctors in the UK are over-smug about the low level of litigation, a point of view expressed forcibly by a correspondent to the *Lancet*, now in the United States, who said, 'I am British, a refugee from a system where the patients were not sufficiently enlightened by the Press or the profession to know when they were being ill-treated, and where physicians were not equipped, through insurance, to satisfy the just demands of a severely abused patient'.[13]

Envoi

Patients are obliged to use a limited repertoire of stratagems in order to retain even a reasonable degree of autonomy in the transaction with the doctor. Those who are lowest in the pecking order have the greatest difficulty. The disappearance of the fee in the NHS has diminished patient power although it has many advantages. The principal and most important of these advantages is the removal of any financial bar to access to medical care. Only those who have lived or worked in societies where ill health threatens not only their future but economic survival, can understand what a boon this is. It has also, in the years of affluence, allowed the development of a first class hospital service which is now beginning to creak because the flow of new capital has virtually ceased. It has altered the balance between patient and doctor, in some senses in favour of the doctor, in another sense in favour of the patient. A number of patients now regard the doctor as their servant: a state employee, employed by them, the taxpayers, to do their bidding. Those who choose to treat their doctors in this way meet with a cool reception and seldom achieve their objectives, although they do provide doctors with reasons for adopting a trade union stance in negotiation.

4 DIAGNOSIS

The Needs and Expectations of Patients

Most people are healthy most of the time and become patients only intermittently and for relatively brief periods. Despite a very considerable literature on health services little attention has been paid to the reasons people come to doctors.

Most people who perceive themselves as ill do not immediately decide to become patients. A number of women in South London, who kept health diaries, recorded an average of thirty-nine symptoms for every one they brought to the doctor.[1] The usual response to feeling ill is to seek advice from parent, spouse or friend and to take some self-prescribed remedy. Proprietary remedies available without prescription are, as a study of television advertising shows, a major industry vying with alcohol, tobacco and cosmetics. A pharmacist in Southwest England sold two items for self treatment for every one dispensed on doctor's prescription.[2]

Symptoms are likely to lead to consultation with doctors if they are sudden in onset, severe, or painful. They are also likely to lead to consultation if they are thought to be serious. Paradoxically, the fear that there is something seriously wrong may act as a deterrent, either because people feel unable to face an unpleasant reality or are afraid of the consequences – especially admission to hospital or the prospect of surgery.

Some of those who are ill refuse to consult because they are not prepared to, or feel unable to, become sick. There is a certain protestant ethic which regards illness as a sign of moral weakness and prefers to deny the existence of symptoms. The self-employed and the small farmer may, in marked contrast to those employed by large organisations whose job satisfaction is minimal, refuse to become sick although patently ill.

Other deterrents to the consultation are the fear of rebuff or the absence of a particular doctor. Patients know their doctors and if they have been rudely received, chastised for calling out of hours or arriving without an appointment, are naturally reluctant to run this risk again without cause. There is still in our society a sense of identification with a particular doctor, 'my doctor', which has survived the organisation of group practices.[3] This relationship, which is seen as special, provides some safeguards against being thought foolish, thoughtless or demanding, and also facilitates communication. Because the doctor knows me as an individual, knows the problems which I face and to some extent the secret parts of my life, he or she, no matter how imperfect, is preferable to a stranger. Occasionally this bond may be a deterrent. Neither those friends who are patients, or their children who identify the doctor with their parents, are likely to be prepared to discuss matters about which there is guilt and shame and may prefer an anonymous stranger.

Underlying the decision whether or not to seek professional help is the consistent sense of being inferior, of being of lesser account, than the doctor. It can be argued that illness by interfering with autonomy causes regression towards childlike dependence and this is certainly true of severe illnesses. Indeed the relationship between surgeon and patient can be seen as that between parent and infant, the surgeon being given permission to handle the body in the most intimate way while the patient remains entirely passive. On the other hand, many of those who decide to become patients are not seriously ill and their needs do not require regression towards increased dependence.

The reasons people consult doctors can be encompassed under these headings:

1 The diagnosis and treatment of disease
2 Reassurance about the meaning of symptoms
3 Help with the problems of living

4 Certification of sickness
5 The prevention of disease

Most people know that persuading doctors to respond to their needs depends upon presenting their case in a way which the doctor finds acceptable. They also know that in practice this means symptoms of physical disease which may be exaggerated or diminished as the occasion seems to demand.

Diagnosis in General Practice

The doctor should be able to tell what is wrong, even if he cannot always be expected to put it right. Doctors share this view of the importance of accurate diagnosis and in our medical schools and teaching hospitals diagnosis is king. It is the first part of the mechanistic model of disease, equally applicable to faulty plumbing, which sees diagnosis being succeeded by treatment leading to cure. Diagnosis consists of attaching a label to symptoms or abnormalities which predicts the future and the response to treatment – this is its usefulness to individual patients.

There are, however, two distinct approaches to diagnosis, a practical approach which does not seek to pursue diagnosis beyond the stage that predicts therapy or outcome, and a theoretical approach that seeks to refine diagnosis to the limits of the possible. Generally speaking the practical approach is characteristic of general practice, does not rely heavily on technology, is cheap and subject to error. Its cost benefit is relatively high. The theoretical approach is less subject to error in physical terms, relies on technology and has a lower cost benefit. It is more likely to add to our knowledge of disease.

Characteristic of general practice is the undifferentiated problem. In attempting diagnosis the first essential is to discover the reason for the consultation. In hospital the assumption, not always justified, is that the patient seeks diagnosis of physical disease and appropriate treatment. This assumption, readily made by young doctors trained in our schools, is never justified in general practice. The reason for the consultation may be reassurance, support, certification of sickness or prevention of disease.

Given that the primary reason is diagnosis of symptoms, the approach used by experienced practitioners is based upon probabilities and the possibility that the underlying disease is life-threatening.[4] Common things are common but there are a number of relatively uncommon diseases in which medical intervention critically affects outcome and a correct diagnosis may be life-saving – for example, acute appendicitis. In the surgical ward appendicitis is a very common diagnosis; whereas most general practitioners, unless they have an unusually large number of children and young adults in their practice, will not see more than four or five cases a year. Many conditions which are common in hospital are seen rarely in practice and conditions which are rare in hospital are unlikely to be seen by most practitioners in a lifetime.

The primary objectives of diagnosis in general practice are different from those in hospital. They are, to exclude serious remediable disease and to achieve a plan of action. Each consultation has to end with a decision, usually made by the doctor and usually involving a prescription. The objective in hospital is accurate definition of the problem, leading (as in general practice) to a management plan. But unless the condition demands an urgent response, decisions about management are usually delayed until the diagnosis has been clearly established. It is considered bad medicine to initiate treatment before this has been done, as treatment may modify the disease and make diagnosis more difficult.

The first moments of a consultation are spent in greeting and establishing some form of relationship which will facilitate communication. Each doctor tends to have a standard ritual for doing this and it can be little more than 'good morning, sit down, what can I do for you?'[5] When status differences are very great it may be even more abrupt. In private practice when a young doctor is trying to create a good impression with a new patient it may be considerably protracted. It is important, and often neglected, because unless a good relationship exists it will be difficult to elicit an adequate history of fears, or of matters which are associated with guilt or shame. One of the strengths of general practice is that such a relationship may have been established as a result of previous encounters and little time need be spent in confirming that it still continues.

Once this first phase is over, the doctor, by a series of questions, investigates the problem. This technique is based upon the rapid generation of diagnostic hypotheses which are then tested and either rejected or pursued. In the case of a young woman who presents with headache and vomiting, the most likely diagnosis is migraine, but meningitis or bleeding inside the skull are both conceivable and serious; both require immediate hospital referral. Initial questions would be chosen to confirm a diagnosis of migraine and to exclude the serious possibilities.

Once committed to this task, doctors are difficult to deflect from the single-minded pursuit of their objective. Deflection may be necessary, especially if they have misunderstood the nature of the presenting complaint or problem. But it may be almost impossible for the patient to intervene successfully until the questioning or history-taking and examination are completed. At this stage the doctor is understandably reluctant to take a deep breath and to start all over again.

When the doctor is satisfied that he has reduced the diagnostic possibilities to a small number, he may or may not proceed to examination. If he decides that some form of examination is necessary, it will almost always be done on a selective basis, it will be carried out to confirm or deny certain diagnostic possibilities, it will not be complete, and he may fail to notice or accept findings which appear irrelevant to the framework in which he is working. He will see what he is looking for but may not notice what is there.

An examination may be carried out, not primarily as a diagnostic aid, but in order to fulfil patients' expectations. It may be a necessary part of reassurance: it is almost certainly unacceptable to tell somebody that their lungs are fine without examining their chest. The doctors' 'triangle' – that area of the chest accessible by undoing one button – is sometimes used to reassure patients: it is quite unsuited to reassuring doctors that hearts or lungs are normal.

At the end of the period of questioning and history-taking, and following whatever examination may ensue, most doctors will have already formulated a plan. Following a brief explanation they will proceed to close the consultation, usually by writing and presenting a prescription. This encounter has a high cost-effectiveness in terms of useful diagnosis. Most serious, acute and remediable disease will have been identified to the point that decisions about appropriate treatment or referral to hospital will have been properly made. In many, if not most cases, no real diagnosis, in the sense of an accurately defined pathological process, will have been achieved but this is of little importance in determining outcome.[6]

Most young doctors entering general practice find their inability to achieve 'respectable' scientific diagnosis very disturbing and in direct conflict with what they have been taught in medical school. A normal expectation of patients is that they should receive a diagnostic label. The patient who replies, when asked what is wrong, 'That is what I came to find out', enlists our sympathy. Unfortunately, attaching diagnostic labels, rather than confessing ignorance, may create mythical diseases. A patient of mine was employed in a factory where his job involved stacking tractor tyres. One day, not surprisingly, he developed a sore shoulder. Referred by the factory nurse to the accident department of a nearby hospital, he had a number of x-rays, which were normal. He was then referred to an orthopaedic surgeon and following further x-rays and a course of physiotherapy, sought an explanation for his pain. He was informed that he probably had 'a touch of arthritis in his shoulder joint'. As he is a young man, this diagnosis is untenable but he has not returned to work as he now has 'arthritis'.

Doctors seem reluctant to confess ignorance but patients do not expect infallibility. The statement 'I do not know', accompanied by suitable reassurance based upon the knowledge of what has been excluded – heart disease, for example – is normally quite acceptable.

In addition to history-taking and clinical examination, family doctors may undertake or order investigations. This is much more widespread in the USA and is much more commonly part of the patients' expectations. Only a very small proportion of new episodes of illness seen in general practice in the UK are referred. Most published figures suggest something under 10 per cent. In my own practice, where I had direct access to the laboratory, radiology and also the possibility of directly admitting patients with non-urgent conditions, the figure fell to 4 per cent. Nowadays most general practitioners have open access to the laboratory and to most, if not all, common radiological techniques. This, coupled with the provision of diagnostic aids such as electrocardiography, should enable doctors to achieve an accurate diagnosis in many cases. Unfortunately, there is much evidence that many practitioners not only lack basic diagnostic equipment but also make little use of pathology or radiology departments.[7] The general practitioner who uses to the full the diagnostic aids available to him is in a position to employ specialists, primarily for their technical skills, and only occasionally requires consultant advice. Patients in these circumstances are admitted either for care or for specific technical procedures of investigation or treatment; for example, bronchoscopy or removal of a diseased gall-bladder.

Diagnosis in Hospital

The majority of patients admitted to acute hospital beds are referred by general practitioners, the important exceptions being those admitted from accident and emergency departments. Because they are referred and have already been screened by family doctors, the content of physical disease of a potentially serious sort is much higher than in the population of patients presenting to general practitioners. Patients whose problems are primarily psychological or who need support or to be sick are under-represented; but if they do present at hospital their real needs may be overlooked. Medical students are taught to collect all the available data and to undertake a complete physical examination. The emphasis is on the physical: social and psychological data are relatively neglected, although awareness of their importance is growing.

The approach of clinicians, particularly those who are experienced, is much more selective but is, nonetheless, less concerned with outcome, seriousness and immediate decision-making than that of general practitioners. In addition to history-taking and examination the patient in hospital will be submitted to investigations, ranging from blood tests and x-rays to exploratory operation. Some of these investigations are undertaken to pursue and confirm a clinical diagnosis, some are routine and may be included as either 'while we are at it', or 'just in case'. Hospitals which have achieved, or seek to achieve, very short lengths of stay for patients tend to carry out a large number of investigations initially, in case they are needed, because ordering them serially in response to earlier results protracts stay.

Underlying this approach is a philosophy that regards accurate diagnosis as an end in itself and a missed diagnosis as the greatest sin. It is also argued with some force and with real justification that it is in this way that understanding of disease can be increased. The disadvantages are of three sorts. The usefulness of any particular investigation is not related to the extent to which a positive result will alter management or benefit the patient. In myocardial infarction the diagnosis is usually clearly established on the basis of a clinical history and electro-cardiographic findings. In addition, as a result of the damage to the heart muscle, the amount of certain enzymes in the peripheral blood is raised. It is almost routine to estimate these enzymes, usually on several occasions, although in most instances the results neither add to diagnostic accuracy nor affect management. Occasionally patients may be submitted to investigations which are unpleasant, or even dangerous, primarily to increase knowledge. Such investigations, it is widely recognised, are only justifiable if they benefit the patient. Sometimes however the justification appears tenuous. Instances, or theoretical possibilities, provide what appear as adequate reasons but they are not always critically balanced against discomfort and risk.

Secondly, investigation may uncover abnormalities whose existence was unsuspected. At first sight this might seem to be entirely beneficial; but in many instances the abnormality is of no significance and in others it is either unimportant or untreatable. A further danger stems from the sheer quantity of information.

> The human mind behaves like an information system of limited channel capacity. Or, to put it more bluntly, we

become easily overloaded with information. As we acquire more and more data we get into a state where we make mistakes, overlook the obvious, and can't see the wood for the trees. What is new and important, is that we are beginning to realise how much doctors' performance (in both diagnosis and management) is damaged by the constant flow of large quantities of (often irrelevant) information in a short space of time.[8]

Lastly, the cost of investigations is constantly increasing, in part because of an increase in their number and in part because of the development of new techniques, such as the CAT scanner, which depend upon expensive and sophisticated technology. The scanner and other recent advances in radiology, for example the development of ultra-sound, have the great advantage from the patient's point of view that they are non-invasive and do not involve distress or discomfort.

Most treatable and curable conditions which are not self-limiting can be diagnosed without sophisticated technology, and in general practice. This includes most infections (many of which are self-limiting), mechanical defects, ruptures, piles, varicose veins, injuries, common endocrine and blood disorders, diabetes, disorders of the thyroid gland, common anaemias and many disorders of the heart and circulation. Sophisticated technology, advances in biochemistry, immunology, and radiology, have added greatly to our knowledge and have improved our diagnostic skills. Their contribution to a reduction in mortality or even to an improvement in the quality of life seems however to bear an inverse relationship to their increasing cost. It is at least arguable that money spent on diagnostic machinery and the people to man and service it would, if diverted to other purposes such as the care of the elderly, make a greater impact on the quality of life.

Cost

There can be little doubt that our society sees diagnosis as something which should be vested in highly and expensively trained doctors. Indeed, dissatisfaction with the diagnostic competence or diagnostic authority of general practitioners often underlies a request for specialist referral. On the other hand, it has been demonstrated both here and in Canada that a nurse, without any special training, can make good decisions about the nature and potential seriousness of symptoms.[9] The only failing of nurses in a Scottish study was that they did not always appreciate the potential significance of minor degrees of chest pain. A cadre of nurses, given a little additional special training, could provide a diagnostic service in the community which would be cheaper and probably almost as effective in the identification of serious or potentially serious physical disease as our present doctor-based service.

At the moment, the view that all our citizens should have access to the most elaborate and modern diagnostic techniques is only beginning to be challenged. The ideal diagnostic technique is accurate (that is, it distinguishes between those who do and do not have the disease), painless, non-invasive, risk-free and cheap. If it does not satisfy these criteria it can only be justified if the diagnosis leads to useful intervention. Generally the profession has encouraged the proliferation of diagnostic aids in an uncritical way and has accepted the philosophy that knowledge is an adequate end in itself. As a result, failure to provide the resources of new machinery is seen as bureaucratic resistance or inefficiency, and an informed debate about the possible choices in spending is only beginning. For a specialist, the inability to provide the best possible is very frustrating. To have to settle for the second rate when trained and motivated to provide the best is extremely difficult. Yet it may be that, given a limited resource, the cost of providing the best, when the number of patients likely to benefit, their age and the extent to which they may be cured are considered, may be too high in relation to other ways of spending the same amount of money. At the moment we lack both the necessary tools to assess cost-benefit critically and a satisfactory forum in which proper choices can be made and implemented.

5 TREATMENT

The need for Treatment

Death is the only inevitable consequence of conception, and in coming to terms with premature death and with disease all societies have found it necessary to seek acceptable explanations. Explanations fall into three categories; retribution by the gods, human failings of omission or commission, or the workings of a blind indiscriminate fate.

The growth of knowledge has not made such beliefs obsolete. Patients still sometimes see illness as retribution, often believe that if they had behaved differently they might have escaped, and may resent what seems to be the workings of malevolent fate.

It is human nature to seek explanations not only for disease but also for recovery. These explanations, which rapidly become beliefs, are based upon the association of phenomena. 'I have lived to eighty because I never smoked/always smoked/ never drank/ate an apple a day/ eschewed fish . . .' By analogy all therapies are effective. We believe in treatment.

Until recently I made a livelihood on the strength of this belief. Many of the conditions I treated were unaffected by drugs, many were incurable, sometimes the treatment was harmful but on the whole it was assumed to be the reason for recovery. Therapeutic nihilism is growing as a result of mounting evidence of the dangers of drugs. An examination of medicine cupboards shows huge amounts of unconsumed medicines. Everyone is aware of the thalidomide disaster. This distrust of drugs has to be considered alongside the huge consumption of self-prescribed medicines.

In brief, we are ambivalent towards treatment with drugs.

Doctors, trained in an environment in which their role is projected as the accurate diagnosis of disease, leading to treatment and cure, are therapeutic activists. When in doubt as to the validity of prescribing, they rationalise so doing as a response to patients' expectations. They generally fail to realise the scepticism with which many patients now regard what sometimes seems to be the inevitable prescription.

Drugs

The assessment of the value of drugs is not easy. It rests most securely on a properly carried out double blind randomised controlled trial. This is a trial which compares the active drug with an inactive placebo which looks the same. Allocation to treatment with the active drug or the placebo is by chance and neither patient or doctor, hence double blind, knows which is being taken. By this technique inactive compounds such as sugars have been shown, not only to alleviate symptoms but also to produce 'side effects'. Furthermore, their effect may be altered or enhanced by changing the colour of the tablet or capsule. There have been few adequate drug trials of this sort carried out in general practice – particularly trials of antibiotics, tranquillisers or anti-depressants in the management of relatively minor illness.

It can be argued in anthropological terms that the placebo effect is in part due to the giving of a symbol by those of high status to those of low status: the prescription is an outward and visible sign of power to heal. In the fairly recent past, the expectation of many was nothing more than the all-potent bottle of flavoured liquid.

Nonetheless doctors too readily assume that treatment is the expectation of their patients. Given adequate reassurance or counsel, many patients, given the choice, will reject a prescription. Much prescribing is effectively placebo prescribing, but no placebo appears as such in the popular formulary, and in practice antibiotics, tranquillisers and many other potent and expensive drugs are prescribed primarily for their placebo effects. This is more likely if the patient expects, as many reasonably do, to be told the nature of the treatment. It is, at the least, difficult to say to a patient, the treatment which is being prescribed will have no effect on your disease but because you expect to be given something to take, it is likely to make you feel better and reassure you that you will recover. On the other hand, it is easy to prescribe penicillin for an infection, even when it is almost certain to have no useful effect.

The implication is that few, if any, commonly employed drugs are used either specifically or effectively. There is a positive relationship between the accuracy of diagnosis and the appropriateness of treatment. When diagnosis is inexact, which is common in general practice, or the patient's need is primarily reassurance, counsel or certification, it is easy to be critical of prescribing.

There have been, however, particularly since the last war, a number of major therapeutic advances. An ideal treatment is a specific response to a specific disorder which restores normality, without any undesirable effects. There are relatively few treatments which satisfy these stringent criteria. The correction of vitamin deficiency before irreparable damage has occurred, for example the treatment of Vitamin B_{12} deficiency, the cause of Addisonian or pernicious anaemia does so. The replacement of hormones when their production is deficient, as in hypothyroidism or myxoedema, is both effective and when the dose is right, virtually free of any disadvantage. The treatment of diabetes mellitus with insulin prolongs life but does not completely correct the abnormality. Penicillin used to treat infections with sensitive organisms satisfies all the criteria in the absence of allergy, but there are few, if any, other antibiotics which are as free from undesirable effects. There are many valuable drugs which while not satisfying the requirement of restoration of normality have both prolonged life and alleviated symptoms. Diuretics, drugs which counteract the body's tendency to retain fluid, particularly in heart failure, and drugs for the control of high blood pressure are examples. Powerful pain killers are of great value in the management of self-limiting conditions or before and after surgery, but are generally much less satisfactory in the treatment of persistent pain.

The pharmaceutical industry has itself pioneered the development of many invaluable drugs and has made huge profits. Some of these profits have been devoted to education and the promotion of research but the cost of drugs remains extremely high. Each general practitioner in the United Kingdom prescribes £15,000 worth of drugs each year and the real benefit of much of this prescribing must remain in doubt.[1] There is very little worthwhile research which provides good evidence of the benefit of the most commonly used medicines, such as sleeping pills, tranquillisers, antidepressants or antibiotics; while some medicines such as cough mixtures have been shown to be virtually valueless.

Mortality

The leading causes of premature death throughout the Western world are coronary heart disease, stroke, chronic bronchitis, accidents and cancers. Together they account for more than eighty percent of total mortality.

Of these, cancer is the only one which offers the prospect of cure. Most people have an unnecessarily gloomy view of cancer. They are usually aware of friends, relatives and acquaintances who have had cancer and who have died. They may be unaware of those who have been cured. Those who are cured do not advertise the fact and many who are cured never knew they had the disease.

It has been argued that most cancers have an environmental origin. Many causative factors are known. Cigarette smoking causes lung cancer and is associated with cancers of pancreas and bladder. Blue asbestos causes cancer of the lung and its lining – the pleura. Exposure to radiation increases the risk of leukaemia and of skin cancers. Cancer of the cervix is associated with multiplicity of sexual partners.

Further evidence for environmental factors derives from the varying incidence in different parts of the world. Many cancers are common in some countries and rare in others. Cancer of the large bowel is common in these islands, rare in most of Africa; cancer of the breast is common here, uncommon in Japan; primary cancer of the liver, common in the Bantu, is almost unknown here.

Chronic bronchitis and coronary heart disease are strongly associated with cigarette smoking. Once these abnormalities are established medicine can offer nothing more than the prolongation of life. Cure in the sense of restoration of normality is no longer possible. Yet the control of atmospheric pollution and cigarette smoking offer the prospect of huge reductions in chronic bronchitis and it is at least arguable that premature coronary heart disease is largely preventable.

The role of diet in the aetiology of coronary disease has been the subject of continuing, and at times heated, debate. It is likely that the mechanisms involved will become much clearer in the near future but many would now be prepared to state that a reduction in the intake of saturated fats coupled with an increase in the intake of fibre and an increase in physical exercise would have a dramatic effect on premature mortality.

Stroke, although also related to disease of the arteries, in this case the arteries supplying the brain, is different. It is commoner in women and generally does not affect younger people. It is associated with high blood pressure but not all those who have strokes are hypertensive. With the exception of a rare form of stroke in young people which is caused by the rupture of abnormal vessels, there is no useful treatment for stroke. Physiotherapy, nursing, and possibly speech therapy are important in obtaining maximum recovery but doctors are much less important than devoted and concerned relations.

Surgery has a place in the management of the congenital abnormalities which cause bleeding around the brain in young people and attempts have been made, with some success, to improve the flow in the major arteries of old people. This is only possible if there are warnings that a major stroke may be imminent and offers little prospect of materially diminishing mortality. A more aggressive approach to the treatment of high blood pressure might have a greater impact but this is not yet proven.

There are many problems in deciding to treat raised blood pressure. It is a contributory factor in causing both stroke and coronary heart disease but there is no certain evidence that lowering levels, particularly when the level is not very high, is beneficial. As a rule raised blood pressure is symptomless so that a decision to treat converts an individual who feels healthy and is not ill into a sufferer from disease. The cost of drugs to treat a single person, even over many years, is not enormous but minor elevations of blood pressure are so common that an aggressive approach to its treatment could, in total, be very expensive. Treatment is not free from undesirable effects ranging from light-headedness or dizziness to impotence.[2] Many patients are well without treatment and feel ill when taking pills. This substantially reduces the possibilities of their continuing to take them. For all these reasons a decision to treat is both major and difficult. It can only be made in the light of knowledge of individuals – their maturity, the absence of neuroticism; and it requires that they understand the benefits and disadvantages and are prepared to tackle the task as a co-operative venture between doctor and patient.

Accidents

Accidents, particularly road traffic accidents, are an important and tragic cause of mortality and serious disability, especially in the young. As in coronary disease, stroke and chronic bronchitis, medical intervention can make little impact by comparison with prevention. One of the commonest complaints made of the medical profession is the difficulty of getting a doctor in an emergency. Accidents are frightening, sometimes horrifying, and it is not surprising that inability to get a doctor causes so much resentment. Doctors are reluctant to respond for a variety of reasons. It can be maintained, not always truthfully, that there is nothing that he or she can usefully do. First aid and prompt transfer to hospital are what is required. As there is little that can be done, it is not justifiable to desert a busy surgery and to inconvenience and to delay so many others. Nevertheless underlying these rationalisations is a reluctance by doctors to face their own fear and feelings of helplessness. Anyone who has worked in practice will be familiar with the knot of unrelieved anxiety that exists between receiving a summons to a road accident and the discovery that the damage is, after all, relatively trivial.

There are other deterrents to attending accidents, including the experience of being the third or even fourth doctor to arrive, and reluctance to become involved in the court procedures which commonly ensue. In one or two places practitioners have organised themselves to provide an extremely efficient, well-equipped and highly competent service for road accidents.[3] In these circumstances accidents are seen as a challenge rather than a disturbing and inconvenient threat.

The surgical and medical management of major and often multiple injuries is complicated and demands a genuine team approach. The experience gained in wartime and in special centres such as the Birmingham Accident Hospital has been put to good use. One of the results of improved management is the survival of patients who would previously have died, some of whom survive to live with permanent and major disability.

Health By The People

Most deaths from coronary heart disease, stroke, and cancer, occur relatively late in life. A sudden coronary death in the late seventies, while one is still active, may be preferable to progressive enfeeblement and dementia.

The major change in expectation of life in the last hundred and fifty years has been due to a reduction in infant and childhood deaths. Most of the improvement is due to better nutrition, better hygiene and immunisation against infectious disease; relatively little is due to curative medicine. In the greater part of the world improvement in health of any considerable degree still depends not upon doctors, but upon having enough to eat and proper drains.

Although it is true that curative medicine has not had a dramatic effect on mortality, particularly in middle age and in the elderly, the number of people living into their eighties has increased. Many of them are seriously handicapped and a high proportion have some degree of dementia, an unhappy word which means nothing more than the loss of full cerebral function. A further improvement in health and a reduction in premature mortality depends, as it always has, not on doctors but on the people. It requires on the one hand individual decisions to stop smoking or to take more exercise, and on the other political decisions to increase taxation on cigarettes or to increase the penalties for drunken driving.

Unfortunately our knowledge of the determinants of behaviour and of acceptable methods of inducing modification is still in its infancy. There is a delicate balance to be struck between legislation that discourages certain sorts of behaviour and legislation that interferes with legitimate autonomy. It is however certain that the contribution of doctors to improved health is largely confined to providing knowledge which individuals or society may choose to act upon or to disregard as they will.

Benefits

The foregoing account of treatment has underemphasised the benefits. Bacterial infections, tuberculosis, syphilis, pneumonia, meningitis and many others have become unimportant causes of mortality and morbidity. Diabetes, thyroid disorders and other endocrine malfunctions can now be controlled. The management of high blood pressure and heart failure has been transformed by the development of new drugs. The advances in anaesthesia have made surgery not only safer but have extended its horizons. It is very easy to forget, or underestimate, the contribution of the surgery of such common conditions as piles, hernias, or varicose veins to the quality of life. The removal of cataracts, the restoration of hearing by fenestration and the successful replacement of osteoarthritic hips have transformed life for many people. Transplant surgery offers hope to those with irreversibly damaged kidneys.

Any attempt to assess the cost-benefit of treatment must take into account the age of the patient and the degree to which the treatment restores autonomy and the ability to work and live a normal life. It must be sensible to devote more resources to saving the life of a child than to prolonging the life of an octogenarian. Unfortunately, some lives can only be saved at the price of disability, but this is a risk implicit in the decision to treat.

There is no doubt that we expect therapy, and expect doctors to be therapists. There is no dispute that the legislation which restricts the practice of surgery to trained surgeons is desirable. There is, on the other hand, considerable disquiet about doctors' use of drugs, and some would challenge their exclusive right to prescribing. Generally speaking doctors have been very responsible in their use of drugs of addiction and the notoriety of the few is a tribute to the probity of the many. It may well be that doctors have been over-cautious in using such drugs for the relief of post-operative and other pain which was either transient or accompanied terminal illness. But to make them widely available on demand is a course that nobody who has seen a heroin addict of twenty could readily advocate.

A substantial reduction in our present drug bill could be achieved if patients and doctors could accept that most ills cure themselves, if doctors could accept that all their patients do not expect a prescription and if patients learned the limitations of the pharmacopoeia.

If the primary diagnosis of disease could be vested in the hands of a nurse, so could the management of minor ills. As has been shown in many parts of the world, a restricted number of drugs can be used effectively by health assistants to manage common problems. Nonetheless, we still need and we can still afford doctors. Doctors bring to diagnosis and treatment something of real value, indisputable in the case of surgery, probable in the management of serious and uncommon disorders, but open to some question in the management of minor and self-limiting disease.

6 REASSURANCE

The Need

The human being in pain is as much concerned with its meaning as its intensity. I suspect and like to think that animals are not concerned with pain as a threat but have only to contain the pain itself. For humans the existence of pain raises a number of questions: is it a herald of death, does it threaten disablement, will it lead to hospital admission or require surgery for its cure? It is not surprising that many people come to doctors seeking reassurance that their symptoms are of no serious significance. Unfortunately they are often disappointed, as doctors frequently fail to provide adequate reassurance even when it is appropriate.[1]

There are several reasons for this failure. One of the most important is failing to recognise the reason for the consultation. Patients will usually begin by cataloguing their symptoms rather than expressing their anxiety. The doctor, in his turn, will respond by asking a series of questions designed to elucidate further the cause of the pain or other symptom. Having achieved a diagnosis he may well proceed to prescribing treatment without ever having discovered the reason the patient came to see him. It has recently been demonstrated that it may be very difficult for the patient to interrupt this sequence and create an opportunity to talk about the real problem.[2] Faced with the complaint of chest pain doctors will immediately launch into a series of questions regarding its situation, duration, intensity, aggravating and relieving factors, all properly directed at determining its possible cause. They seldom ask 'Why did you come to see me?' – although the answer 'I thought it might be my heart is more informative than the answer to any other question. It immediately defines the problem as anxiety about the meaning of the pain and enables reassurance to be directed at the proper target; it may also predict the nature of appropriate investigation. There is little point in trying to reassure patients they they have not got cancer of the lung without a chest x-ray or that they have not got heart disease without at least examining their heart and probably arranging for electro-cardiography.

It may not always be easy to identify specific fears: patients are still sometimes reluctant to express their dread of cancer or may be ashamed to speak of the possibility of venereal disease. Unless these problems are brought into the open, reassurance is doomed to failure as it will be directed at the wrong target.

Reassurance frequently fails because the doctor, conscious of the limitations of his knowledge, hedges his bets. All too often the statement that 'there is nothing to worry about,' is qualified by 'but I would like you to take these pills – have an x-ray – see one of my colleagues'. Extensive and inappropriate investigations which are negative, or uncover unimportant and irrelevant abnormalities, are self-defeating. If the results are negative, the patient is ultimately forced to one of two conclusions; either 'they' still do not know what is wrong, or 'they' are not telling the truth.

A good doctor must be prepared to live with uncertainty and to carry this burden for his patients rather than to transfer it onto their shoulders. One of the disadvantages of litigation against doctors is that it makes them much more reluctant to behave in this way.

There are some doctors who by being alarmist and attentive get the best of both worlds at the expense of their patients. Such doctors on hearing a few noises in the chest may diagnose pneumonia, and having created unnecessary alarm, visit twice a day until the patient has recovered. If their diagnosis is at fault and the patient becomes worse or dies the doctor will have been seen to have done everything possible. If the patient recovers, the doctor has snatched them from the jaws of death by his skill and concern. Many people have been unnecessarily converted from health to chronic invalidism by the ignorance and timidity of their doctors.

Communication

An almost universal complaint about doctors is 'They don't tell you anything!' Sometimes patients' reasonable questions regarding their disease or its treatment are interpreted by doctors as challenging their authority. This is such a common experience that they will often preface their questions with phrases such as, 'I hope that you will not think me foolish but . . .', 'I am so sorry to bother you but . . .'. The environment of hospital does not encourage the exploration of fears which may appear foolish and which are hard to articulate and doctors unaware of their existence are unlikely to be successful in allaying them. Effective reassurance depends upon recognising the need and answering the need in specific and appropriate ways. Patients must be given the opportunity to express their fears and the opportunity to ask questions.

One of the reasons for complaints about communication is that information, sometimes very detailed information, is transmitted at a time when the patient is unable to receive, comprehend or assimilate it. If a patient is told in an outpatient department that he needs to come into hospital and this news is unexpected, he will fail to retain any information conveyed during the remainder of the consultation. Their need to assimilate and deal with the consequences of an anticipated hospital admission preclude their attending to whatever else is said, no matter how important it may be.

Reassurance, in order to be effective, must be directed at the proper target, must be based upon proper grounds and must be provided by a proper authority. Doctors' authority rests in part upon their expert knowledge, in part upon their sacerdotal powers, or role as father figures. Many patients seek referral to specialists as a court of higher appeal, reassurance given by practitioners being seen as not based upon adequate knowledge. Doctors may be reluctant to respond to such requests for two reasons. First, such a request challenges, in a very direct way, the doctor's authority and it requires considerable maturity to respond to such a challenge without emotion or without attempting a defence. Quite often a compromise is reached which denies the possibility of immediate referral but allows it as an option if recovery is delayed. Secondly, practitioners may, with good reason derived from experience, be sceptical that referral for reassurance will achieve its objective. Sometimes inadequate communication between doctors does not make it clear that the reason for referral was reassurance; and sometimes, lacking the family doctor's knowledge of the psychology of the individual, the specialist may find it very difficult to resist the temptation to investigate the matter further, thereby running the risk of making reassurance impossible.

Faith

People still speak of having faith in their doctors. Faith is founded in part upon authority and in part upon experience. A practitioner who has a continuing relationship with a family may inspire faith which derives from the family's past experience that his judgements and prognostications were proved to be right in the past and are therefore likely to be right in the future. This faith tends to be vested in an individual and is not transferable to colleagues, especially those who are more junior, or to specialists whose right to faith may appear more rationally based. This is one of the principal advantages of a personal doctor and one of the main arguments for a continuation of primary care based upon general practice. Such faith, which is a firm base for reassurance, is more likely to be vested in the old rather than the young and its absence adds considerably to the burdens of those starting a career in general practice. My first grey hairs were welcome as evidence that no longer could patients complain that I was too young, and I could henceforward regard remarks about my youthfulness as complimentary rather than denigratory.

Nurses cannot in our society replace doctors as sources of reassurance because they are not vested with comparable sapiential authority. This is not to say that, both in hospital and within the community, they do not provide valuable and valued reassurance which stems from their experience and knowledge, but to point out that this will often have to be reinforced by the status that a doctor possesses. I find it much easier to conceive of a nurse replacing the practitioner in the diagnosis and management of physical disease than as replacing him as a source of effective reassurance.

Reassurance is an important and neglected part of the doctor's role. Patients often come to doctors seeking reassurance, and their need is often unmet because it is not recognised – or, if recognised, because the response is inappropriate.

7 PROBLEMS OF LIVING

Isolation

Ivan Illich used the phrase 'those who have difficulty in living with the human condition' to describe some of those who seek the help of doctors. There are three main reasons why they do so. First, the doctor may be seen as representing sapiential authority, as a surrogate parent. Secondly, many are persuaded that such states as being anxious or sleepless are an expression of abnormality or disease and are not tolerable when they can be relieved or 'cured' by appropriate drugs. Lastly, the doctor is the route by which a number of benefits, some social welfare payments or improved housing may be obtained.

Most of those with problems in living are characterised by isolation. Successful living is dependent on emotional security, on being loved, on being wanted. Man is a social animal; solitary confinement is among the most destructive of punishments.

Society is organised on the basis of groups, or in sociological jargon collectivities; whose size varies from the very small, the family, to the very large, the nation. Every group is characterised by a set of values, which is in a sense absolute, and from which derives a number of beliefs, or norms, about right and wrong and that which is acceptable or unacceptable. Membership of a collectivity, or group, depends upon showing acceptance of its norms by behaving in an appropriate way. Members are disciplined by ridicule, disapproval, ostracism or in the case of nations by imprisonment or even death. Those who are most vulnerable are those who belong to only one collectivity. It has been shown that many of the women in Clerkenwell, judged by the criteria used by psychiatrists, are depressed.[1] In this study depression was associated with low social class and significant protection was afforded if the women had one other person with whom they had an intimate relationship or if they were able to go out to work. Among the advantages of education and high social class is the possibility of membership of many groups. Men are more likely than women to enjoy multiple membership and are thereby less likely to suffer isolation.

Those who have most difficulty in living successfully are those who depend upon a single source of support: failure of that support is a crisis. The vulnerable include those who have recently left home, the bereaved, single parents and the elderly. Immigrants characteristically join others from similar environments and while this creates ghettos in our large cities, it also affords significant protection from what would otherwise be intolerable isolation. The young woman who has moved away from home to live with husband or lover, particularly if the decision involved some degree of disagreement in the family and a sense of rejection, is at great risk. This risk is increased if she is tied to unsuitable housing by small children. In these circumstances even minor marital disharmony may produce feelings of intolerable isolation and may lead to self-poisoning, as a cry for help, or less commonly to a more serious suicidal attempt.

There has been in the last few years a very sharp increase in the number of people deliberately taking overdoses of drugs. Those who successfully commit suicide by means of drugs are characteristically male and elderly. They frequently take care that they will not be discovered and their suicide notes are concerned with important matters such as where the car keys may be found, reminders about the insurance and the location of their will, rather than eloquent and moving messages of farewell. By contrast those who take overdoses and who seldom, but sometimes, kill themselves are young and mostly female. They have often declared their intent and will usually ensure that their action is suspected or known.[2]

Students who are living away from home for the first time, and find identification with the values and behaviours of peer groups difficult are also in danger. Those who have been at boarding school may be at an advantage in that while they can have problems in making new friends, they have been through the exercise before and are used to coping with homesickness.

Bereavement can be contained in a supportive community. I recently accompanied a friend to the funeral service of her husband. Although neither she or her husband were conventionally religious, the size of the congregation, which represented to her an act of corporate love by a large number of people, was a source of comfort. The smaller size of families and the considerable mobility in our society make it increasingly likely that the bereaved may be denied the comfort of children:

> formal mourning with all its helpful ritual seems restricted more and more to the important public figure or to the ethnic minorities. Usually the cadaver is whisked away, often to a damp and ill-lit annexe to the undertaker's premises little deserving of its grand title of the Chapel of Rest. The routine cremation service is an anonymous occasion for decorum giving no place to tears or memories, or it may interfere with the next funeral. The ritualized grieving of the Jews, the alcoholic celebrations of the Irish wake, or the baked meats of the old-fashioned funeral seem vastly superior to the present anaemic and untherapeutic routine. This sets the scene for a grieving that is furtive and unshared. We do not wear black or take much time off work. At the end there is for most of us neither a bang nor a whimper. This naturally intensifies the emotional reactions of bereavement.[3]

Retirement removes the daily support of colleagues or work-mates, and the widower has been shown to be unlikely to live as long as his married contemporaries.[4]

Unhappiness

Quite apart from those who may be categorised as being at particular risk of becoming isolated, most people at one time or another face difficulties in their marriages, or their work, and have to cope with bereavement and disappointment. The usual response is unhappiness of variable intensity and duration which may or may not be accompanied by anxiety. Unhappiness is associated with feelings of tiredness, of things requiring too much effort, failure to work or study effectively, loss of appetite, diminished libido and sometimes disturbance of sleep. Psychiatrists regard these symptoms as those of depressive illness. Within the category depression they recognise two main varieties – reactive when the depression appears to be a reasonable, although abnormal response, to external events and endogenous, when there seems to be no adequate explanation. In practice the distinction is blurred and may reflect nothing more than a description of two ends of a spectrum. Generally, more serious depressions in older people are more likely to carry an endogenous label. The natural history of both is recovery after a period of time, usually measured in months, but during the acute phase both carry the risk of suicide.

Practitioners have been slow, because of inadequate training, to recognise that the symptom of tiredness usually indicates depression. Thanks to better training, postgraduate courses and the advertising of drug houses, somatic symptoms which are associated with depression are increasingly recognised and huge amounts of anti-depressant drugs are prescribed. In the present state of knowledge it is reasonable to regard endogenous depression as a disease, which may have a genetic or biochemical cause although that cause is unknown, and to prescribe appropriate treatment. For every patient who presents in general practice with symptoms of endogenous depression there are many who come to the doctor with symptoms which are attributable to their unhappiness or to their difficulties in 'living with the human condition'.

Anxiety labelled as anxiety neurosis or sleeplessness labelled as insomnia may come to be regarded as diseases instead of a normal human response to the problems of living. Hypnotics, tranquillisers and anti-depressants accounted for 16.5 per cent of all drugs prescribed by general practitioners in England in 1970. This represents 40 million prescriptions, virtually one prescription for every man, woman and child.[5] To regard these people as diseased, as suffering from reactive depression, and to respond to their need by prescribing drugs is to perpetuate a state of illness. Money will be spent to provide pills and those who take them may function at less than their full potential. Many will become psychologically, and a few physically dependent on drugs. Most seriously of all, such a response implies that unhappiness is a disease that is amenable to medical treatment.

Personal Care

An alternative response to those who seek the doctor's help in living is possible. It rests on providing emotional support when needed and in assisting people to work out their own solutions. One of the strengths of general practice is that doctors tend to remain in practice in the same area for most, if not all, their professional lives. This creates an opportunity for continuity of care over a long period. It also allows the doctor to acquire a considerable knowledge of the community in which he works, its values, its idiosyncrasies and the interrelationships within it. The community also knows its doctors, their strengths and weaknesses. This is most obvious in small stable communities and clearly is less applicable to those parts of large towns where there are many transient residents. The relationship between doctor and individual patient or family is built up, by means of a series of brief encounters over the years, into something of considerable importance. It may be enriched by a sense of things shared, of crisis, of illness, of birth and of death. This can provide a secure basis for emotional support which can best be described as mutual love.

This does not imply a state of continual dependence leading to ever increasing demands. People, even those with major continuing problems, need to become patients only intermittently. Nevertheless at times when problems can no longer be contained, a familiar figure, with whom there is already established a personal and secure relationship, is readily available. Indirect evidence that this is important and valued is provided by the resentment that has been freely expressed about deputising services, impersonal rotas and rigid appointment systems which diminish the chance of seeing one's own doctor. It is recognised in the definition of the Royal College of General Practitioners which speaks of '*personal*, primary and continuing care' as the role of the doctor.

Personal care implies a relationship between patient and doctor at a level that transcends technical competence in the sense of skilful plumbing. It has both advantages and dangers. The advantages derive from improved communication and mutual knowledge and trust, the disadvantages from the creation of mutual dependence. Not only are patients dependent on their doctors but doctors on their patients. In fee-paying societies they depend on patients for their income; in all societies they depend on patients for the maintenance of their self-esteem. Thanks to Michael Balint, awareness has grown that the transaction between doctor and patient is as much concerned with the doctor achieving his objective as with the patients achieving theirs.[6]

Dependence implies perpetuation of a child/parent relationship and precludes health, which implies independent adult autonomy. Both parent and doctor require to be needed; unless they feel needed their 'raison d'être' is substantially diminished. Doctors, like parents, find it difficult to accept that their continued attention and treatment are inimical to health.

Often the relationship between doctor and patient is tinged with sexuality and this, if contained, mutual and recognised is not necessarily harmful. If it is not mutual, particularly if the doctor does not recognise it in himself, it is dangerous and destructive. At some time or other most doctors will have had patients 'fall in love' with them. Given time and no encouragement this can be overcome and replaced by a different relationship but sometimes the only useful approach is to refuse to see these patients. Such a refusal should follow a discussion of the relationship: bald rejection may have serious consequences.

Dependence is of two sorts, which may frequently overlap. A person may be maintained unnecessarily and for prolonged periods as a patient, the implication being that they have not yet achieved health and the right to full autonomy. If health is the successful adaptation to disability, continued attendance at surgeries and out-patient departments may reinforce people's perception of themselves as abnormal or unhealthy and encourage 'sick-role' behaviour. This is particularly likely in the case of long-continued or incurable diseases. One of my favourite patients had severe rheumatoid arthritis which she ignored as much as possible. Her friends persuaded her to see a distinguished rheumatologist in Harley Street and I was happy that she should do so. She returned from her visit to London and, with a wry smile, told me that what she had received for her fee and the travelling expenses involved, was a booklet entitled *How to Live With Your Rheumatoid Arthritis*. The rheumatologist's reputation was deserved!

People with high blood pressure, diabetes, and heart murmurs are at risk of being maintained by their doctors in a dependent role. The doctor is unconsciously motivated towards doing so in order to satisfy his need to see himself as useful and busy and sometimes in order to ensure his livelihood. There is an underlying and genuine dilemma in that adequate surveillance of those under treatment for such diseases as diabetes, hypertension or hypothyroidism demands regular attendance. It is very easy for doctor and patient to tacitly agree that the illness constitutes a continuing diminution of full health, and thereby prevent the patient from living successfully and sensibly with their disability.

Even more common is the cultivation of emotional dependence. Those who are isolated and loveless and have problems in living may need a father figure. If the need is temporary, the doctor may be doing a useful and important service by providing emotional support. If the need is continuing, and if the doctor does not recognise his own need to be loved and the extent to which dependence bolsters his own self-image, he may unconsciously allow emotional dependence to become fixed and so preclude recovery and restoration of health.

Nevertheless there are people who are 'incurable' in the sense that it is impossible for them to obtain from other sources the emotional support which they need. I have to believe this in order to justify the number of my own patients who become, to some extent at least, dependent. Such people can be maintained by relatively infrequent but regular contacts with their doctor. If the contact is regular, problems will usually be contained until the next visit or consultation is due. If the contact is haphazard each new problem is likely to result in an immediate and often inconvenient call for help. Many people, especially the elderly, can as a result of regular, once a fortnight, once a month, injections of support, be enabled to live more successfully than if they were left entirely to their own devices. Although this perpetuates some degree of dependence it is useful and important.

8 COUNSELLING

The Need

In a society that is supportive there is no need for doctors to take on the role of father figure. Support from others creates a climate conducive to problem solving. It is part of everyday experience that a long walk with a friend, talking out a problem, is helpful. This was nicely expressed in one family I knew, who whenever faced with a crisis or unhappiness used the phrase 'go climb a mountain', and usually did. Without the contribution of physical exercise, which itself seems to restore a sense of proportion, talking it out can both allow new perspectives and reduce problems to manageable size. The role of the confidant in these circumstances is usually limited to encouragement and lending a willing ear, and this is all that is required. Sometimes the confessional can serve a similar purpose. At the other extreme lies professional psychoanalysis and somewhere in between lie counselling techniques. In all these instances the intervention of others is a help, not in imposing solutions but in encouraging their generation.

Doctors are committed advisers and bad counsellors. It has been shown that consultations in general practice almost always contain directive advice.[1] Indeed part of the patients' expectation is that they should receive advice and if it is not forthcoming will frequently ask such questions as: 'Should I go to bed? Should I eat normally?' There are two problems about giving advice. First, if the advice is unacceptable it will not be followed; and secondly, there is a considerable temptation to give on inadequate grounds advice which may be inappropriate or harmful. Many doctors seem to feel that their responsibility ends when they have delivered themselves of whatever advice seems appropriate: it is then up to the patient to follow it. Failure to act on advice is termed non-compliance, and non-compliant patients are 'bad'. An alternative, but uncommon view, is that the doctor's responsibility should extend, when he or she is certain of their ground, to ensuring that advice is followed. This may mean nothing more than elaborating the reasons why it is important that pills should be taken regularly at a stated time but it may mean using a technique that will encourage the patient to take a decision to diet or give up smoking.

Non-Directional Behavioural Counselling

Non-directional behavioural counselling is a technique seldom employed by doctors, largely because they are unaware of its existence and have not mastered the necessary skills. As with most skills, aptitude varies but most people can learn its use. In essence it is an attempt by the counsellor to help the counsellee to define his problem and subsequently generate his own solutions. In practice adequate problem definition usually generates obvious solutions and it is unnecessary to devote much time or energy to answers.

The art of successful counselling lies in encouraging the counsellee to take his problem out of hiding and define it for himself in real terms. One of the characteristics of those who have difficulty in living is that their difficulties are seen in terms of 'if only'. 'If only I had a better house, a better job, a different husband, less children.' Many people, including both doctors and social workers, are tempted to respond to the 'if only' at its face value and try through social agencies to provide more money, alternative housing or new jobs. As Andrew Malleson has pointed out, such symptom relief no more cures the disease than Valium cures anxiety.[2]

The objective of counselling is to prevent the counsellee from escaping the problem by flight into the fantasy of 'if only'. If a marriage is foundering, a decision must be made as to whether the problem is 'my marriage is at an end', or 'my marriage is in difficulties'. If a job is unsatisfactory, a decision must be made as to whether the problem is 'I can no longer tolerate the present position', or 'I can't find alternative employment.' Counselling is not, as many doctors seem to think, giving advice in a still small voice. Advice such as, 'If I were you I would leave your husband', no matter how gently given, is arrogant in its assumption of the knowledge of what is best. Doctors sometimes give advice such as 'you should change your job, or move house' with very little regard to the economic, psychological and social effects of such actions. Unfortunately the advice may be taken, as people prize their health and aspire to longevity, and are prepared to make major sacrifices in the cause of prolonging life. Prolonged life is not an inevitable consequence of the recommended action and the price may be much too high to pay for dubious advantage. A counselling approach does not preclude an honest statement of the benefits and disadvantages of certain actions but it precludes decision taking by the counsellor.

Such an approach is particularly suited to problems that involve moral or ethical issues. Most would believe that the doctor has no right to impose his own moral standpoint on his patients. In sexual matters he should be able, if his knowledge is adequate, to state the risks of therapeutic abortion or the risks associated with any contraceptive method – the decision should remain with the patient. A counselling approach allows patients to express their fears, to access expert opinion as they require it and so facilitate their decision making.

Counselling is not supportive: it is an attempt to get the counsellee to confront the real nature of the problem. It is normally good practice to arrange the consulting room, where the doctor's role is usually supportive, so that the patient sits at the side of the desk. In this way eye contact can be avoided and patients can be comforted or reassured by touch.

Eye contact is a phrase which derives from behavioural science. As a general rule when talking to people we do not look them 'straight in the eye'. We occasionally steal glances in order to discover from their facial expression how they are reacting to what we are saying; but we will only look them in the eye if we wish to stress that something is important or wish to dominate. Those used to authority will seek to dominate by staring others out and will so arrange things that supplicants have to sit at the other side of an imposing desk. The outcome of many social encounters, from securing the attention of waiters to falling in love, is determined by eye contact. A switch from a supportive to a counselling role demands some degree of confrontation, and doctors changing roles will draw back their chairs and seek eye contact.

Support has to do with phrases and noises such as 'tch tch', 'dear, oh dear', 'how awful for you'. Counselling uses such words and phrases as 'So?', and 'what do *you* think you should have done?' It is somewhat aggressive as its aim is to prevent the person who is being counselled escaping into fantasy, into 'if only' land. Because of this it is not a suitable technique to use on one's family, who find, as I learned from experience, such confrontations uncomfortable, and coming from a husband or father intolerable.

In order to be effective, counselling must be concerned with the real problem, not with the problem as first presented. Real problems involve the emotions. Counselling that fails to produce evidence of 'gut feeling' is unhelpful, and has not been successful in making counsellees confront the nature of their difficulty. Evidence of emotion derives from 'non-verbal cues' (another phrase used by behavioural scientists), which include not only facial expression but tone of voice, attitude, ways of sitting, fidgeting and the use of eye contact. The counsellor must seek to keep the patient's attention on the subjects that he or she finds uncomfortable and would seek to avoid. Because of its aggressive and uncomfortable characteristics it may be wise for the doctor to return to a supporting role before the session ends in order to provide evidence of continuing care and concern.

It has been argued that such a technique is very time-consuming and quite unsuited to the exigencies of practice and the six-minute consultation. This would be true if counsellor and counsellee were meeting for the first time and it was necessary to establish a relationship as a prelude to progress. It would also be true if the objective of each session was a problem completely defined, acceptable solutions agreed and decisions made. It is not true if a good relationship already exists and if the objective is not a package neatly tied with blue ribbon, but rather new perspectives which can be taken away, considered and possibly applied to the problem. A smaller number of relatively brief sessions separated by time may be much more valuable than a single lengthy encounter because the intervals allow new ideas to be tested against the realities of the situation.

The Role of Others

Professional support is not the sole preserve of doctors, and the social worker is increasingly cast in this role. This emphasis has disturbed those nurses who work in the community as district nurses or health visitors, and who have for many years provided, in addition to their nursing skills, an amount of support and care that has received little in the way of public recognition. One of the major problems surrounding the concept of the team in general practice is the jealousy with which individuals protect their special relationships with patients. These relationships gratify a need for love, sometimes as strong in the professional as in the patient. If this is recognised it may be used by patients to manipulate the situation in their favour. To be involved with social workers, to need them, is in some degree stigmatising and there are few people in the higher social classes who would accept counselling from a social worker. The status of doctor or psychoanalyst is a necessary precondition of their acceptance.

Those of us who have learnt by painful experience the importance of human relationships in the doctor-patient transaction may be in danger of inflating their significance. Some of my students have complained, not without justification, that their concept of general practice derived from my teaching excluded the diagnosis and treatment of disease. It does, however, seem that the rewards I derive from the practice of my profession stem much more from helping people through their problems than from treating their diseases and I am therefore tempted to see this as a central part of my role as a doctor. As one of my colleagues expressed it, 'The most rewarding thing that I do is to help a young couple achieve a satisfactory sexual relationship. I can then say, I need never see you again. I really feel that I have done some good.'

A utopian society would support its members and would

have no need of doctors to help people 'live with the human condition'. This underlies some of Illich's appeal and the fantasies many people have about life close to the land in small village communities. Nevertheless until society becomes a utopia and so long as doctors are readily available, people will come to them seeking help with problems which have nothing to do with disease in the sense of recognisable pathology. If we continue to base our health service on doctors as the main source of first-contact or primary care, then they must be trained to recognise those symptoms which stem, not from disordered function, but disordered relationships. They must also be taught useful responses.

9 SICKNESS

Sick Role

Disease may be defined as the existence of pathological abnormality: illness as the presence of symptoms. Disease is objectively determined, illness is subjective. Sickness, on the other hand, can be considered as a socially sanctioned state. Those who are regarded as sick are, on the one hand, excused their normal obligations and on the other entitled to certain privileges which extend from lying abed to substantial sums of money.

As Talcott Parsons first pointed out, society demands of those who choose to be sick that they behave as sick people.[1] If they are to be excused normal obligations, they must forfeit the privileges of the well. They may not plead sickness to escape work and then go to a football match: such behaviour is seen as malingering. The sick are expected to wish to get well and to give evidence of this wish by behaving sensibly, by taking appropriate medicine and in the case of an illness that lasts more than a few days by seeking the doctor's help.

By no means all those who are ill choose to become sick. The self-employed are less likely to do so, as are those who feel that others depend upon them or that they are indispensable. In some families it is assumed that minor illness is 'tholed' – that is, borne without complaint. One of my children, when young, caught his finger in the car door. Receiving what was quite clearly inadequate sympathy he complained, 'You're only happy if I bleed.'

Serious or obvious disease has the advantage that there need be no dispute about the right to become sick. When the illness is not obvious and there are no easily detectable outward and visible signs, others have to be persuaded that the illness is genuine. In my own family the ability to push the mercury in the thermometer above normal is a very important part of proof. If you cannot continue to run a temperature, you are unlikely to be allowed to be sick.

When the illness is minor, most people would prefer to be half-sick: that is, to be excused things they do not enjoy. The ploys used in this situation deserve the attention of a Stephen Potter. They include the 'domestic martyr', who, despite what is clearly anguish, insists on creeping around the house doing unnecessary chores, making everyone else uneasy and unhappy. The only effective counter-ploy is 'well if you say you're alright, I'm off'. The problem is that unless the disappearance is permanent, the martyr is placed in an even stronger position, when the escapee eventually returns. Such games are usually transient but occasionally can become a destructive way of life.

The doctor is involved in two ways. He is involved in attempting to cure or alleviate the presumptive disease and he is also required to confirm that the illness is genuine. There are many people who wish to obtain the advantages of being sick in order to avoid their obligations: to escape going to school, going to work or having intercourse. Such people come to the doctor not to be made well but to be confirmed and maintained as sick.

Sickness Absence

Those who work for large or impersonal organisations, whose job satisfactions are minimal and who see themselves as unimportant cogs in a very large machine, are motivated to become sick with little provocation. Sickness absence is growing in industrial societies and is not the result of an increase in disease but to altered behaviour. In organisations that make provision for a number of days sick leave on full pay, this may be seen by employees as an entitlement to additional annual leave and is almost always used in full. The nature of the work may influence the amount of sickness; it is not surprising that working at the coal face is associated with high absence rates.

Trade unions have been successful in diminishing the likelihood that sickness will lead to losing a job but in some occupations fear of dismissal may still be a deterrent from becoming sick.

The doctor plays a key role in legitimising sickness: society demands that he distinguish the malingerer from the genuinely ill. In practice this is a totally unreal expectation and he has virtually no option but to endorse the individual's decision to be sick. Before doing so certain rituals are almost universal. The patient does not come to the doctor in the first instance with a naked request for a certificate of unfitness for work, although that is commonly the only reason for the consultation. A man who has a hangover on Monday morning and decides not to go to work will present to the doctor symptoms of headache, or stomach upset. The doctor, even if he knows that the reason is a hangover, is tempted to respond to the symptoms by attaching a diagnostic label such as gastritis. Once this decision has been made he can continue happily, as the patient now has a disease and it becomes appropriate not only to issue a certificate but also to prescribe treatment. The patient returning home with certificate and bottle of medicine can now expect sympathy and special consideration rather than castigation for his drunkenness.

Because there are no objective means of assessing subjective phenomena, especially pain, it is almost impossible for a doctor to establish that a patient is malingering. Malingering – that is, feigning symptoms in order to avoid work – is rare. Maximising trivial symptoms in order to justify work avoidance is common. Once the doctor has agreed to issue a certificate and to prescribe treatment any sense of guilt is effectively removed and the individual has legitimate and adequate reasons for becoming sick. Cheating the system is becoming socially acceptable and those who can simultaneously claim sick benefit and work as private entrepreneurs are envied and admired rather than regarded as dishonest.

As in many instances being sick causes little if any economic hardship, the number of people continuing to work is more surprising than the number who choose to be sick. The only effective pressures counteracting the tendency to become sick for trivial reasons are a personal ethic which regards illness as a sign of weakness or the disapproval of family or peers. Volvo, by making a small group of workers responsible for the complete assembly of a car, rather than for a simple repetitive task, have reduced sickness absence. This may be due to a feeling that their absence lets down the team and so must be seen by fellow workers to be fully justified.

Certification

The doctor's position is extremely weak. Occasionally refusal to certify is successful but doctors are reluctant to engage in such direct confrontations. Persistent refusal is one of the reasons why patients change doctors, who, aware of this, sometimes rationalise the giving of certificates by stating that if they don't, somebody else will. Probably the most useful response by the doctor is to make the patient responsible for the decision not to work and, unless there are valid reasons for doing so, avoiding statements such as 'I think you should be off work'. The best response to 'When do you think I will be fit to go back to work?' is 'When do you want to return?' Some firms have abolished certificates for short periods and absence has diminished rather than increased. A certificate in respect of even transient illness tends to mean at least a week off work.

As many as 100 million National Insurance Certificates may be issued each year, most of them by general practitioners. This amounts to something between four and eleven certificates a day for each doctor. A third of the population claims at least once each year and about 320 million days are lost each year through illness.

There is a positive side to the doctor's role when, as is occasionally the case, an individual may be endangering his health by continuing to work. Such instances are, however, relatively uncommon and the much commoner problem is that of encouraging and persuading those who have been ill to return to work. Being sick rapidly becomes a habit and it may be very difficult to give up the privileges of the sick and to resume normal responsibilities.

The Sick Housewife

Those who are not employed – particularly women – who

wish to manipulate their environment by being sick, cannot obtain a certificate that excuses them washing dishes or sexual intercourse. In this circumstance the bottle of pills symbolising treatment, being 'under the doctor' or 'attending the hospital' are necessary as proof of the entitlement to be sick. Many people obtain repeat prescriptions over long periods with minimal or no contact with their doctor. If this situation is challenged, the doctor may be surprised to find that his statement 'I don't think that you need to continue with these pills' is not welcomed but stoutly resisted. This has been interpreted as psychological dependence; often it is an expression of a continuing determination to be sick. If the doctor remains adamant, the patient will offer alternative symptoms and in the last resort will change doctors. Armed with the bottle of pills it is possible to plead inability to fulfil whatever obligations are distasteful.

Occasionally the sick role can be used constructively: both Florence Nightingale, after her return from the Crimea, and Charles Darwin chose to become sick in order to escape the duties that otherwise would have been thrust upon them. Cabinet ministers, generals – all had to visit Miss Nightingale and she continued to exert considerable influence from her bed or chaise longue. Darwin, by being sick, created the time to write *The Origin of Species*.[2]

Many people come to doctors not to be made well, but to be kept sick. It is not surprising that a transaction in which the two principals have such different objectives is often unhappy. This conflict is almost never discussed. Instead both doctor and patient go through a series of rituals at the end of which the patient achieves his or her objective and the doctor remains unhappy and dissatisfied. Since doctors are very unsuccessful in using certification to protect society, it is not difficult to argue that they should no longer be required to certify incapacity. A major reduction in sickness absence can only be achieved by improving job satisfaction, by providing financial disincentives, or recreating a sense of crisis and of mutual interdependence such as occurs in times of war. It is difficult to be loyal to a huge state organisation or a multinational corporation if one's place in the hierarchy is near the bottom, and hard to believe that one's absence will affect the function of the whole.

Doctors do not always recognise, because they have not been taught, the importance to many people of the 'sick' label and too readily assume that sickness is synonymous with disease. Their role in legitimising sickness will always be unhappy because not only does it conflict with their self-image as people who cure disease, but provides almost no satisfactory objective criteria by which they can make decisions.

10 PREVENTION

The Need

Prevention is popular in theory but neglected in practice. In the past the major emphasis has been upon the control of infectious disease. In the developed world it has now shifted to reducing premature mortality from diseases of middle and old age, the smoking diseases, lung cancer, chronic bronchitis, coronary heart disease, other cancers and stroke. In the world as a whole malnutrition and the consequent mortality from infections including parasitic diseases remains the major problem. The last century has seen a dramatic decline in the number of deaths from infectious disease in infancy and childhood. This has been mostly due to improved nutrition, housing and hygiene. Specific immunisation and antibiotics have played a part but the major reduction anteceded their development.[1] Life expectancy at birth has increased dramatically: in contrast, life expectancy for the middle-aged, especially the male, has only increased by a relatively small amount.

I have on a number of occasions invited groups of senior medical students or general practitioner trainees to outline their conceptions of their role. Invariably the prevention of disease is not mentioned or is introduced as an afterthought. This reflects the priorities in medical education.

Nonetheless there are a number of well recognised preventive activities that are regularly carried out in general practice and that patients seek. The most obvious of these are immunisation and routine antenatal care. Immunisation of infants and children on a large scale is relatively recent. The first successful mass programme was immunisation against diphtheria, which began in the 40s and has almost eliminated the disease. This was followed by the inclusion of tetanus and the now controversial whooping cough to create what became known as the 3-in-1; three injections of which are given to infants between four to six months and one year of age. To this was added poliomyelitis, originally as an injection, and now as an oral dose of living attenuated virus. Measles vaccination is becoming routine and schoolgirls are offered the opportunity of immunisation against rubella (German measles) in order to protect them against the possibility of infection during early pregnancy. Vaccination against smallpox, if successful in the first instance, always produces a reaction and since smallpox seems to have been almost, if not entirely eradicated from the world, is no longer justified. Immunisation against tuberculosis by the injection of BCG (Bacillus Calmette-Guerin), an altered form of tubercle bacillus, gives partial immunity only and is probably not justified except in the case of those, such as doctors and nurses, who are at special risk. To this already long list must be added immunisation against specific diseases for those who travel, either to protect themselves or to meet international requirements. These include cholera, yellow fever, typhoid and paratyphoid A + B. Finally, vaccines that provide protection against known strains of influenza are also available and valuable in protecting the elderly and those with chronic bronchitis.

The techniques of immunisation are simple and doctors in the United Kingdom increasingly delegate the task. Such delegation appears sensible but diminishes the possibility of a dialogue about the desirability of the procedure. At the moment parents would certainly expect to be persuaded and reassured before agreeing to whooping cough vaccination. Another disadvantage of delegation is that it prevents the doctor using the occasion of the immunisation to enquire about an infant's progress, to allay fears and to educate.

The advantages and need for antenatal care are well recognised and there are very few women who do not present themselves to the doctor during the early months of pregnancy. Good antenatal care combined with improvements in the management of labour and the care of the newborn, especially the premature, has reduced perinatal mortality: but this reduction has been achieved at the price of making pregnancy a disease.

An important aspect of preventive medicine is family planning. This, together with therapeutic abortion, has created, probably for the first time, a new sort of relationship between doctor and patient. The relationship is new because doctors have generally agreed that in this instance their role is to carry out the patient's wishes, to respond to the patient's demands. They may still advise that the pill is not the most suitable contraceptive or that abortion is not justified, but having expressed their reservations, usually accede to the request. The patient effectively controls the transaction.

Screening

Because many diseases, some of them serious, are symptomless for long periods of time, attempts have been made to identify affected individuals before symptoms occur. A screening procedure is an investigation, test or examination which, applied to a 'healthy' population, identifies correctly those who have the disease. A screening procedure should not need to be carried out by doctors and should be usable by nurses or other health workers. In addition to identifying the disease correctly, a satisfactory procedure must be relatively cheap, and must be acceptable to the 'patients' or subjects. The disease must be fairly common and most important of all it must be possible to do something useful about it.[2] There are very few screening procedures that satisfy these criteria. Screening newborn babies for phenylketonuria (PKU) and other inborn errors of metabolism is cheap, requiring nothing more than a drop of blood, and successful early diagnosis offers the possibility of preventing serious mental handicap. The only drawback is that the abnormality is uncommon.

The cervical smear (or 'Pap' test) is often undertaken by doctors as part of routine post-natal care, or in the course of vaginal examination primarily undertaken for some other reason. This is more properly 'case finding' rather than screening. As a screening procedure it has the disadvantages that it is not always acceptable, particularly to those at greatest risk, it is not particularly cheap, and most seriously it is not always clear what action should be taken in the face of minor abnormality which does not amount to the existence of a cancer. Most evidence available at the moment would suggest that an intensive campaign to encourage women to be screened will reduce mortality from cancer of the neck of the womb, but that the cost is high.[3]

Screening middle-aged populations for diabetes mellitus is cheap, simple and acceptable but is of little value because there is no evidence that treating mild symptomless disease does any good.

Mass miniature radiography (MMR) had a place when tuberculosis was widespread: it is of little use in the detection of cancer of the lung because the results of treatment are so bad.

Because early diagnosis of cancer of the breast is associated with better results from treatment, there have been attempts to devise satisfactory screening techniques. All these suffer the limitation that early diagnosis, while increasing the successes, by no means provides a guarantee of cure. In America many women have been taught and use the technique of self-examination. In the United Kingdom nurses have been trained to examine breasts, and mammography, a radiological technique, has been used on an experimental basis. Mammography has the disadvantage that the doses of radiation are not negligible and if repeated might themselves induce cancer. All these approaches, including thermography, identify many lumps which are not malignant and many of these have to be biopsied. The extent to which biopsy and focusing attention on the importance of breast lumps creates unnecessary fear and anxiety is a matter of opinion.

Doctors have the opportunity to use contacts with patients to 'case find': that is, by undertaking such activities as recording blood pressure or testing urine even when these do not seem to be immediately relevant they may discover symptomless disease. In addition they can, from their knowledge of personal and family history, identify individuals at special risk. In the United Kingdom most people see their family doctor at some time in every five-year period. It is therefore theoretically possible to discover almost all those with unusually high blood pressure without mounting any special screening procedure.[4]

The 'check-up'

The 'health-check' has had a considerable vogue in the United States and has been sold in the UK to higher business executives on a commercial basis. It has recently come under heavy fire as another 'rip-off' by the profession because most of the abnormalities discovered, at considerable cost, are not amenable to treatment. A request for a check-up may be a cloak for specific anxieties about the meaning of minor symptoms. To the mechanistically minded the check-up provides reassurance that things are in good going order and gives permission to continue the same life-style.

Doctors in Britain who have no financial inducement to respond to the request for a check-up tend to be unenthusiastic. They will often rationalise this reluctance as doubt about the cost-benefit of the exercise and as fear of producing neuroticism or hypochondriasis.

The preventive measures which would reduce premature mortality are well known. They include legislation to make the wearing of seat belts compulsory, rigid enforcement of speed limits, improvements in vehicle and road design and effectively preventing those who had been drinking from driving. The drunken pedestrian is also at high risk.

If cigarette smoking were to stop, there is no doubt that lung cancer, which has been steadily increasing, would begin to diminish and would ultimately become rare. Coronary heart attacks and sudden death in the middle-aged would be much reduced. Chronic bronchitis would become an uncommon disease. The experience of the medical profession, which has largely given up smoking, shows these expectations to be justified.[5]

Attitudes to smoking, particularly in the higher social classes, have changed. Smoking first became fashionable among upper-class men, gradually percolated downwards through the social classes and then involved women. It is not unreasonable to predict that smoking will now begin to diminish in our society and that it will be almost unheard of in fifty years' time. During this time millions will have died unnecessarily young.

Major changes in our diet which would reduce the amount

of saturated fat and increase the content of polyunsaturated fats and of fibre would not only reduce deaths from coronary disease but might also diminish the incidence of large bowel cancer, of appendicitis, of diverticular disease of the colon, of piles and possibly of varicose veins.

Changes of this sort have far-reaching effects. Stopping smoking would create unemployment, threaten the economies of tobacco-producing countries and remove a substantial source of government income. The evidence that alterations in our diet would reduce premature mortality from ischaemic heart disease is steadily accumulating and has been shown in Finland to be effective on a community basis.[6] A marked reduction in our consumption of animal fat and an increase in our intake of polyunsaturated fats and of dietary fibre would threaten the agricultural industry. On present evidence governments could justify removing subsidies on butter and subsidising certain margarines but would find it impossible because of the effects on the economy.

Those who escape death during their working life are likely to live on to die slowly. Many of them in the process will become enfeebled and demented and require a great deal of care over long periods of time. At the moment we are unable to meet the demand for services for the elderly: successful reduction of premature death would make this imbalance worse.

From the point of view of the economist, concerned solely with financial implications, sudden death, unattended by the medical profession, on the day of retirement from productive work offers the most advantageous economic solution.

Health Education

One of the panaceas often suggested for the world's ills is a major investment in health education. The purpose of health education is not, as it is often seen to be, the transmission of knowledge, but altered behaviour. The knowledge of the dangers of alcohol has not prevented drunken driving, or the risks of promiscuity, venereal disease.

Altered behaviour depends upon individual decisions made in response to a number of factors of which knowledge o the risk is only one. More important than risk is the need to conform with the norms of the collectivity, group or society in which people live. Disapproval by family or peers is much more likely to have a significant effect than a degree of added risk. Children's smoking habits derive mainly from their parents, partly from their siblings and peers.[7] The welcome increase in the number of non-smoking areas in trains and aeroplanes, no smoking in theatres and the growing number of restaurants prepared to impose some limitations all exert pressure on the smoker.

Extra risk, the initial effect of the introduction of the breathalyser, or the experience of having had a coronary, can often tip the scales, but lesser degrees of risk, especially if the effects will not be apparent for years, as in lung cancer, have little or no effect on behaviour. The young have little interest in longevity and it is much more important to them that they should respond to the pressures of the moment. It is sad that the young, who hazard much, run risks, while the old, who can afford to live dangerously, decline to do so.

The doctor in his contact with patients has the opportunity to educate. Doctors have in their training been subjected to a great deal of didactic teaching and when they wish to educate tend, predictably, to adopt this style. Unfortunately this is the style which is least likely to achieve the objective of altered behaviour. Behaviour is not arbitrary, it is the outward manifestation of values which are deep seated and which can only be changed slowly by an alteration in the individual's perception of her or himself. In order to stop smoking the individual must perceive himself as a non-smoker: he must begin to dislike himself as a smoker and ultimately find it intolerable that he should continue. A form of non-directive counselling is much more likely to facilitate behavioural change than didactic advice. The only exception is when, under favourable circumstances such as a recent heart attack, the patient can legitimately be frightened into believing that continuing to smoke is as risky as walking the tightrope over Niagara. An open-ended, non-didactic approach has the advantage that specific deficiencies in knowledge or misconceptions can be identified and sometimes corrected.

There are a relatively few well established preventive

measures which are well known to the public and in which the doctor has a clear and useful role. Apart from these, any major advance in preventing premature death rests with the individual and with society as a whole. It would be possible for government to take decisions which would improve the health of the middle aged. Such decisions would have major consequences for the economy. Health is no longer a matter for doctors; health is in the hands of the people.

11 CARE

Caritas

Doctors are expected to care. They are seen as belonging to one of the caring professions. This title has emerged because other descriptions of nurses, physiotherapists, occupational therapists and medical social workers – professions ancillary to medicine, for instance – were seen as demeaning. The isolation of caring as the common characteristic is interesting: presumably it is not a feature of law or accountancy.

Care is a word with a multitude of meanings ranging from the caritas of Paul's famous epistle to the Corinthians to the custodial function of borstals. Caritas, charity, love. I wonder to what extent these words are now associated with the public image of doctors. Charity has been diminished by its dissociation from love, or even from concern, so that it is seen as little more than the giving of alms to ease an unruly conscience or in response to successful begging. This is a pity because as caritas, enshrined in the motto of the Royal College of General Practitioners 'Cum Scientia Caritas', or as St Paul used it, it expressed love freed from eroticism. Compassion in some ways suggests Lady Bountiful or at least an unreciprocated emotion, immediately associated with looking down.

A doctor who is to be directly involved with patients must like the human race. It is easy to hate the human race in large impersonal numbers, for example communists or football crowds, but difficult for many not to identify with an individual in trouble. If a doctor is to be effective as a communicator, if he is to earn the trust which is the basis of reassurance, if he is to provide comfort, he must do more; he must love his fellow men and women. Loving others is touching lepers, restoring to every man his right to human dignity. It is not paternalism, it is identification.

The Nature of Care

Doctors talk increasingly about the quality of care. They are usually referring to audit, to ways of examining input, process and outcomes in the management of disease – a legitimate, proper and valuable exercise, but little to do with care in the sense of concern for individual human beings. A modern hospital, either built or derived from buildings designed to care for the sick poor, is a fine place to undergo major surgery or intensive care during a life-threatening illness. It is a poor place in which to be ill, to convalesce or to die. The erosion of privacy, institutional food, the impact of nursing schedules, noise, the routine sleeping pill are all accepted with wry humour as being a necessary price to pay for the privilege of treatment. They certainly ensure that most short-stay patients aspire to return home at the earliest possible moment.

Those who are ill require rest, the possibility of sleeping during the day. They need to withdraw into their private cocoon and to remain insulated from the outside world. One of the advantages of hospital admission is that it provides an effective barrier and a protection against the intrusion of ordinary day-to-day affairs. If being in hospital does not involve feeling ill, as is often the case, this isolation from normal concerns can be very irksome. The tycoon will rightly insist upon a telephone by his bed and daily visits from his secretary. In addition to rest and treatment those who are ill, as part of their regression into dependence, need comfort. Not only does the sick child need the comfort of its mother, but adults the comfort of those who love them.

The nurse is still cast in her traditional role of comforter. One of the sadder things about hospitals is the extent to which they make it difficult for relations to provide comfort. This was nicely expressed in an article, the source of which I have long forgotten. The author described the experience of visiting his sick child in hospital, his wanderings along interminable corridors, his difficulties in stopping any of the many people who passed him in order to ask the way, they all seemed so preoccupied with some urgent and important task. Eventually he found the ward and timidly pushed aside the formidable doors to be met by a nurse, who bustling starchily towards him asked without preamble, 'What do you want?' He went on to contrast this experience with visiting his friendly neighbourhood police station where on entering he was greeted by the constable behind the desk with a smile and 'Good morning, can I help you?' Those visiting hospital find the atmosphere chilling and feel themselves unwelcome intruders. There is a sense that they will somehow interfere with some essential and life-saving task. I remember vividly as a medical student wishing to enter an operating theatre but feeling that my unheralded entry would put the surgeon off his stroke with some disastrous result: it was as if I was to burst into the billiard room when the world champion was about to pot the black.

A close friend accompanied her mother, who had had a coronary, to the hospital. They were received in the accident and emergency department and she and her husband were excluded while an increasing number of doctors, students and nurses and various pieces of equipment disappeared behind the screens. After what seemed an eternity, the most senior doctor emerged to tell her that her mother was dead. No one had thought that she would have wished to be with her mother, or that her mother would have wanted the comfort of her daughter's presence. The only recognition of the human dimension was provided by a coloured student who, delaying momentarily at the tail of the disappearing retinue, touched her arm and said, 'I am so sorry'.

The need for children in hospital, particularly toddlers, to realise that their parents have not deserted them is now widely recognised. Sometimes mothers can stay with their children and in many units visiting is unrestricted. Hospitals also recognise the special position of those who are close to death and make considerable efforts to allow relations to stay for as long as they choose, or are able. But the need for comfort is not confined to the very young and the dying.

Comfort is not distracting chatter, platitudes about recovery or statements about the life hereafter. Comfort is the presence of someone who cares: comfort is the warmth of another body in the same bed. It has much to do with touching: in our society in which direct human contact is so often seen as threatening either sexual or physical assault the nurse is one of the few people permitted to touch. This permission is granted as part of her role as a mother substitute. To most of us the idea of similar permission being given to a male nurse is less immediately acceptable. All the doctors I have most admired have been unafraid and unabashed in their use of touch in providing comfort.

Care is sometimes seen as being antithetic to cure rather than complementary. Until the advent of antibiotics cure of infectious disease depended upon natural resistance aided and reinforced by care. It is difficult to measure the contribution of nursing or a quiet mind to recovery but there is some evidence that their importance may be seriously under-rated. Trouble taken to explain the nature, consequences and likely immediate effects of surgery has been shown to hasten post-operative recovery and to diminish complications.[1] Doctors have largely delegated their responsibility for physical care and have neglected the contribution they can make to emotional care. In the acute hospital once investigations have been completed and therapy begun, agreed or finished, the objective of doctors is transfer or discharge. Their perception is that their responsibility is diagnosis and treatment rather than care and that once their responsibilities to attempt cure have been discharged they need not be directly concerned with care. Because of the doctors' position at the top of the hierarchical tree, their attitudes to patients who no longer seem to be in a position to benefit from curative medicine tend to be adopted by the rest of the staff, including nurses.

Nurses

Nurses, as we know them, are inheritors of the Nightingale tradition; mother substitutes, of impeccable moral standing, devoted to caring for the unfortunate sick; the sick, who have as a result of illness, or wounds, found themselves dependent and far from home. Adult infants who need their bottoms and their noses wiped, to be loved, scolded and sometimes disciplined. To this tradition there has been gradually added the concept of the nurse as a professional: someone who has been trained and is the possessor of a special corps of knowledge and skills. Degree courses for nurses in addition to the diploma of state registration (SRN) have been initiated in at least two universities, and more are contemplated. Nurses are expected to be technically competent and many now carry major responsibilities, especially in intensive care units. The recent administrative reorganisation has meant that few senior nurses have continued to be involved directly in patient care. The ward sister, rich in years and experience, the scourge of probationer and medical student, has largely disappeared. The vacuum left by the involvement of nurses in high technology, teaching and administration, is partially filled by the state enrolled nurse (SEN), a lower order of nurse confined to the more menial aspects of looking after patients. As nurses tend more and more to see themselves as technical assistants making a contribution to the scientific cure and management of disease, it is increasingly difficult to recruit nurses to care for those with incurable diseases, particularly the enfeebled and demented elderly, the mentally handicapped and those who suffer from chronic mental disease.

Caring for those with incurable conditions, particularly those who are incapable of responding normally to affection or love, is demanding. The demented, the mentally handicapped and some of those who are suffering from schizophrenia are incapable of the normal responses of saying thankyou or of expressing their feelings of gratitude in non-verbal ways. They may be difficult and occasionally aggressive. In addition, those who care for them never have the satisfaction of seeing them restored to normal health and must be content with the knowledge that they are doing something useful and valuable for which they are receiving minimal rewards and little recognition. The quality of care in our long-stay institutions may be more remarkable than their much publicised shortcomings.

The doctor's importance in long term care derives much more from his status than his professional skills. The mentally handicapped need love and special education, not medicine. We have, however, chosen to regard their disability as a health problem, a choice which is an accident of history, not a deliberate act. As a result doctors and nurses are seen as the appropriate people to provide care, although the importance of others, especially educationalists, is recognised. A doctor in charge of such an institution is to a considerable extent an administrator. As an administrator he is sometimes helped by the status of his profession, but he is unlikely to have administrative gifts. He has little to contribute in a medical sense to his patients.

Who Should Care?

Our hospitals were founded to care, not to cure: to care for those who could not care for themselves and who had nobody else to care for them. By degrees caring has become a professional activity carried out in an institutional setting. Unless care requires a high degree of technical competence, or skills, it does not need to be provided by trained or professional staff. Love is not a product of training or exclusive to those who hold degrees. The best place to be cared for is at home: it may be the best place to be born; it is certainly the best place to die.

The emphasis on caring as a professional skill and as something provided by a beneficent state has had undesirable results. It has led many people to question their fitness to care. This is particularly true of those who are faced with caring for somebody who is dying. One of their great, and frequently expressed fears, is that their care should be inadequate, that without professional training they are incompetent. It is far more important for patients that their emotional needs are met than that their nurses should be professionally skilled. Providing a small amount of professional help, visits by the doctor and nurse, coupled with encouragement and support and the knowledge that if things get too bad admission to hospital can be arranged, allow the possibility of caring. This is not only so for those who are dying, but for many who are incurably ill.

Doctors sometimes make the mistake of giving prognoses in too hard and too definite terms. Many people are prepared to accept the responsibility of caring for the terminally ill: they have to face bereavement when sentence of death is passed and having worked through this, are ready to accept responsibility for care. If the prognosis they are given is over-gloomy, they will find coping for nine months when they had expected to carry the burden for a much shorter time hard to bear. On the other hand, having faced the fact of death, if death happens sooner than expected, this provides a welcome release.

Too often, hospital admission is seen as a last resort, a final and irrevocable step. Particularly in geriatrics there is a much greater recognition of the role of the hospital as a crisis solver and a holiday home. Short term admissions, before those who are providing care have been stretched to breaking point, can enable them to continue. It may allow them to have a holiday or to cope with other crises, such as illness, in their lives. Very often, unless relief admission is planned, a crisis admission brings home to relations the extent and real nature of the burden they have been carrying, and they will be very reluctant to take the patient home. Hospitals, general practitioners, nurses and relations seldom seem to achieve a team approach to the problems of care, each agreeing to play an appropriate and different part in the light of changing circumstances.

Apart from feeling that care may be beyond their competence, many people also feel that the provision of professional care makes their contribution superfluous. 'If there are homes, if there are hospitals, why should we do it? That is what they are there for, that is what they are paid to do.' The growth of services provided by the state also diminishes local voluntary effort. Philanthropy is seen as a function of the central exchequer funded by taxes rather than as an expression of individual concern for neighbours. The possibility of restoring a sense of individual responsibility, of recreating a caring community, has been diminished by the development of centrally financed social services.

To what extent caritas can be purchased, taught or cultivated remains a critical question. Fathers may care more than plumbers.

12 OLD AGE

The General Practitioner's Role

More and more people are living into old age. The numbers are not reflected in life expectancy figures because of the large mortality in middle age, but those who reach 65 or 70 are much more likely than they were to live on into the eighties and nineties. Those who require long-term care are predominantly female, the female:male ratio being of the order of 3:1. There are two main reasons for this. First, women live longer than men, childbirth has now become safe, and they smoke less. There may well be other reasons for their longevity but these are not clear. Secondly, it is still usual for women to marry men who are older than themselves, and this was even more pronounced fifty years ago, when the present generation of old people married. As a result, widows greatly outnumber widowers and are left to live without the support of a spouse.

It is often said that children are no longer prepared to look after their ageing parents, that respect for parents has diminished. This has sometimes been portrayed as a disintegration of moral standards. While it is true that our society and our culture pay scant homage to age (how often do we hear reference to wise old men or women, as compared with references to silly old fools?), there seems to be little evidence that children are, in fact, less willing to accept the burden of caring for ageing parents. Other changes in our society have diminished the likelihood that they will be able to do so. Not only is the size of families smaller but the number of unmarried children, especially daughters, is much less. Furthermore, the chance that children will continue to live near their parents has diminished.

As a doctor I have been far more impressed by the sacrifices children have made to look after their parents than I have been impressed by their disregard. The presence of an elderly infant in a household can, by the demands for care and the need for constant supervision, destroy the quality of life for a whole family. It may make holidays impossible, it may preclude husband and wife having time together alone and may create tensions in the household which have an effect on all its members.

The problems of old age tend to be multiple rather than single. Reduced mobility due to osteoarthritis, or to more easily remediable disorders such as corns and bunions, coupled with failing sight and hearing, transform minor tasks such as housework and shopping into major undertakings. Falls are no longer trivial accidents but likely to lead, especially in women, to broken wrists and, more seriously, broken hips. Social contacts are diminished, in part by not being able to get about, but also by the death and enfeeblement of contemporaries. Paradoxically those who are becoming deaf are often intolerant of noise and failing sight may make reading either difficult or impossible.

Minor degrees of urinary incontinence are common and the resultant problems of laundering clothes and bed linen, of protecting chairs and dealing with smell are quite disproportionate to the seriousness of the disorder.

Leaving aside physical diseases, such as failing hearts, chronic chest disease, enlarged prostates and cancers, the most serious problem of age is failing mental powers. Some degree of failure of memory, especially for recent happenings, is almost universal. In minor degree this means nothing more than predictable responses to given cues, the same often told reminiscence, but it may well result in the endless repetition of the same question no matter how often an answer is provided.

One of the results of being unable to recall recent events is a sense of being out of touch, of being unsure about things in general. Initially this is most distressing and is often followed by unjustified suspicion, amounting sometimes to paranoia. Things which are mislaid have been stolen, things which have been misunderstood are seen as deliberate attempts to mislead. It is easy to overlook the extent of mental failure and the casual caller, even the doctor, nurse or health visitor, may be deceived by outward appearances. The true extent of the failure may only become apparent if hospital admission or some other move to a different and strange environment becomes necessary.

Adaptation to the new or the unfamiliar is difficult and an almost obsessional preoccupation with the routine tasks of living becomes not only a bulwark against the intrusion of change but also a raison d'être. As a practitioner, I soon learned that routine visits to the elderly should be scheduled to happen on an agreed day and at an agreed time. It was not sufficient that I should drop in when passing. If for any reason I was unable to keep our appointment or was late, this created a major crisis in their lives.

In terms of useful medical intervention the routine visiting of the elderly, which was such a large part of my professional life, is difficult to justify. While it is true that most of these patients, probably all of them, were on some sort of continued treatment with drugs, our meetings were not primarily concerned with their diseases or their treatment. It is probably true that my supervision of their physical health left much to be desired, that I seldom examined them adequately and must often have failed to diagnose even obvious abnormalities. Nonetheless, the relationship was valued by both of us and seemed to make a real contribution to the quality of their lives. The evidence for this rests mainly on their distress if I was not available or if I had, for any reason, to let them down. They would sometimes refuse to see my partners, preferring to wait, occasionally unwisely, on the grounds that only I understood them. This dependence can be seen as unhealthy but if the doctor/patient relationship is to be a personal transaction, rather than an impersonal exchange, it is to an extent inevitable. Old people, like children, are ill equipped to deal with the unknown and feel threatened by strangers. It can be argued without great difficulty that providing emotional support to the elderly is a waste of doctors' expensively acquired skills and many doctors do not readily see it as part of their role. Doctors have the advantage that they are seen by their patients as having a right to intimacy because they are vested with authority to a degree not shared by nurses or social workers. In a general practice which provides continuity of care these relationships develop slowly over the years. Doctors grow old alongside their patients and older doctors have older patients: young doctors are seldom acceptable on the same terms as their seniors to the elderly.

Routine visits, legitimised as the need for the doctor to review therapeutic regimens, can provide a bulwark against total isolation and this is one of the reasons that they sometimes become such an important part of people's lives. Voluntary organisations also make a considerable contribution, and backed by modest state funding provide an economic service. Meals-on-wheels is more than food; it is contact with other people. Churches are important as they give the opportunity for regular meetings with others. The high average age of most congregations represents the threat of isolation as much as either tradition or the imminence of death.

Institutional Care

No matter what sacrifices families are prepared to make, no matter how sophisticated the community care services or how caring the neighbours, an increasingly large number of the elderly require long-stay institutional care. This still remains, however, only a small proportion of all old people. Providing the full range of community services – home helps, home nursing, meals-on-wheels, laundry and occasional transport to hospitals, day centres or church services – can prove to be extremely expensive. Keeping people out of hospital is not always sound economics.[1] Sheltered housing and welfare homes provide an alternative to institutional care. They have two major advantages: they allow the patient to retain some degree of autonomy and their staffing costs are less than those of a hospital. Their staffing costs only remain low if the old people are able, by and large, to look after themselves. That is, they are ambulant, can feed and dress themselves and can largely attend to their own toilet needs. If they become ill or confined to bed, the staff may no longer be able to cope.

Many old people require admission to hospital, most of them for relatively acute conditions. A recent survey in a group of acute general hospitals in Dublin showed that while the over 65s constituted only 11 per cent of the population, they were responsible for 22 per cent of admissions and over 40 per cent of bed days. The elderly tend to stay longer in hospital, in part because of the nature of their diseases, strokes and cancers for example, and in part because so many of them live alone or with aged spouses who cannot accept them home to convalesce. As a result, many hospital units which pride themselves on achieving short lengths of stay, which are busy and which have significant waiting lists for admission, may be very reluctant to admit the elderly, and effectively discriminate against them. The old are seen as not requiring the high technical skills which are available, as being incurable, and therefore more a reproach than a challenge, and as 'blocking' beds which could be used for more important and valuable purposes. This rejection by the prestigious staff infects both medical students and nurses who may come to view caring for the old as a second rate and unrewarding occupation. Nonetheless, most old people who are admitted to hospital are admitted to acute wards, for the management of acute illnesses, and remain in hospital for relatively brief periods. In relative terms the number who require long-term care is small but because each of them may require care for years rather than days, the impact on services is quite disproportionately large and is growing.

Largely because of the reluctance of most doctors to become involved with the long-term care of the incurable and old, geriatrics has emerged as a specialty. It differs from other specialties in that there are few, if any, diseases which are peculiar to old age. By contrast there are many diseases which are peculiar to children and which can be seen to justify paediatrics as a separate discipline. The problems of old age are different chiefly because they are so often multiple and because of the importance of social factors in determining management. Most acute illness in old people which needs hospital admission is dealt with not by geriatricians, but by appropriate specialists. Once the operations or investigations have been completed and the crisis has passed, geriatricians tend to become involved, not to exercise their medical skills but to facilitate arrangements for continuing care. In addition, many general hospitals now have assessment units. These units, which are under the care of geriatricians, accept both direct admissions and referrals from other hospital departments. Their purpose is to assess the needs of old people, a difficult task because of the multiplicity of problems and their inter-relationships, to make a management plan and to initiate appropriate treatment.

It is almost impossible to find a recent report concerned with health services which does not make reference to a multidisciplinary approach. This, together with ritual references to the allocation of greater resource and improved education, makes these reports generally predictable and boring. In the case of geriatrics it is almost justified and one of the ways in which geriatricians so often help their colleagues is by their ability to mobilise appropriate help from a wide diversity of sources.

The population of patients which require long term care is predominantly female. They require care because they can no longer fend for themselves or because they have become too heavy a burden on their relations or spouses. By definition most of their disabilities are incurable. Characteristically many of them are demented to some degree. Dementia is an emotive word which in a medical sense means nothing more than some degree of global mental failure and may range from relatively minor disorders of memory to total disorientation, double incontinence and complete dependence. Almost all of them have defects of sight or hearing: cataracts are almost universal, and many are deaf. Few are fully mobile and many require either assistance with walking or the help of a walking aid. Minor degrees of incontinence are common and disabling. The more enfeebled and particularly those who are demented require not only help with dressing and toilet but may also need to be fed.

Because dementia is common some of these old people find themselves in psychiatric hospitals. The decision as to whether they are cared for in mental hospitals or in other institutions sometimes seems to be more a matter of chance than of rational planning. As their problems stem from degenerative processes, psychiatric medicine has little to offer except to those who are also suffering from depressive illness. There is no doubt that many old people are depressed. But as a rule their depression is completely understandable as a normal response to their situation, and it seems both unnecessary and unhelpful to categorise this as illness. In terms of planning how best to provide care, patients should be classified by need rather than by diagnosis. Mental hospitals are important in caring for the ambulant wanderer. These are the slightly confused active elderly who still bustle about and may hazard not only their own lives but constitute a fire risk to their neighbours. They also provide a more suitable environment for the volatile, quick tempered, still physically powerful and occasionally paranoid old men who may from time to time throw things about or lash out with their sticks.

The needs of those who are no longer able to live independent lives are by no means always similar. There is a world of difference between a woman whose intelligence has been preserved, who is continent but whose mobility is severely restricted, and her bedfast, incontinent, severely demented sister. So long as mental faculties are preserved, the goal of those providing care must be that patients retain autonomy, a sense of individual identity and the opportunity to make the maximum use of their remaining faculties and powers. Unfortunately, this is difficult to achieve in an institutional setting. Institutions must of necessity have rules and rules and regulations inevitably limit freedom. Many of the rules are to protect the old people from accidents. If the staff believe that a fall and a broken hip reflects badly on the quality of their care, they will tend to restrict activity in order to reduce the risk. Sometimes the price is too high: it may be worth chancing a fall to be able to breathe fresh air, to see the clouds and to sit in the sunlight. A sense of individual identity depends in part upon the exercise of autonomy but it also depends upon being able to surround oneself with a few personal possessions, a place of one's own. Single rooms furnished from the houses and flats which have been sold are ideal but they are expensive and they make supervision by staff more difficult. Old people need help but too often help consists of doing things for them rather than helping them to do it themselves. It is much quicker to dress somebody or to feed them than to help them to do it themselves. So doing encourages dependence and precludes rehabilitation.

The proper care of the bedfast and the incontinent requires nursing skills: the care of the feeble elderly requires sympathy, patience, tact and consideration. In some ways it is unfortunate that the care of the old has become so firmly entrenched as a medical responsibility. Doctors have relatively little to offer which derives from their knowledge of medicine. The use of drugs, particularly sleeping pills and tranquillisers, should be kept to a minimum. Unfortunately the need to look after people in wards makes noise or restlessness at night a communal, rather than an individual problem and sedatives sometimes have to be used. Routine visits are important to check physical well-being and to monitor drug treatment but they can be relatively infrequent. The importance of the doctor – be he practitioner, physician or geriatrician – is that he supports the staff. Because of his status, his enthusiasms and concern (or lack of it) are major determinants of morale, the attitudes of junior staff and ultimately the quality of care.

Because of its low content of medical skill, the relative impossibility of cure, the lack of either tangible reward or recognition, geriatrics has been neglected by doctors, and many nurses, especially the young, find it unattractive as a career. A recent report by a Royal College of Physicians Working Party points to the difficulties of recruiting doctors to the specialty and suggests that many more physicians should accept responsibility for some long-term care.[2] One of the difficulties is that in so few places are long-term facilities provided as an integral part of or even near to general hospitals.

Improved care for the old depends upon a recognition of their needs and a decision by society to accord these needs a high priority. When resource is limited it tends to be directed to the care of the acutely ill and to those conditions which are deemed to be curable. The present position is likely to deteriorate even further because the population of the old is going to increase in size over the next twenty years. Maintenance of the status quo, without any improvement, will involve expenditure.

Geriatrics does not appeal to doctors because cure of old age, or even its ailments, is not often possible. It is in a sense unfortunate that the care of the old is seen as a medical problem. Medical and nursing skills are important but their contributions to well being are strictly limited.

13 PSYCHIATRY AND OBSTETRICS

Psychiatry

Psychiatry and obstetrics, apparently odd bedfellows, are differentiated from other medical specialties in that it is at least questionable that their major concern is with disease. Much that is labelled mental disease may alternatively be viewed as deviant behaviour.

Mental illness is different from physical illness in that it threatens individual identity. Those who are legless, armless or eyeless can still demand and expect to be treated as themselves, as autonomous and responsible adults. Those who are categorised and stigmatised as mad have forfeited this right.

The care of those who are severely disturbed has a custodial aspect which is in direct conflict with caritas. Institutions which have to care for aggressive and dangerous psychopaths are frightening to visit and most difficult to work in. The nurses, of necessity mostly male, have to act as wardens and this makes their relationship with their patients extremely difficult. The custodial aspects of psychiatric care were brilliantly and cruelly portrayed in the film *One Flew over the Cuckoo's Nest*: it would be only fair if somebody were to portray with equal insight and sympathy the plight of the custodians.

Mental illness is different from physical illness in other ways. The most important is the relative lack of objective criteria for diagnosis. Laing and others have made and overstated the case that the distinction between mental health and disease is entirely arbitrary. Few doctors, or indeed relatives, can conceive of schizophrenia simply as deviant behaviour, and most of us would believe that treatment which allows a return to living in society is desirable.

Lacking objective criteria for the diagnosis of disease it is possible to define it as a condition for which there is effective treatment. This has considerable practical usefulness. There is also an advantage in labelling as a disease conditions where the patient benefits from being entitled to be sick. By this definition the patient should benefit by being labelled sick. A corollary of being diseased and sick is that the problem becomes appropriate for doctors and other professionals rather than one which requires solution by the individual.

The usefulness of this oversimplification can be illustrated by the concept of alcoholism as a disease. The conversion of drunkenness, a sign of moral weakness, to alcoholism, a disease, is relatively recent. The advantages are almost self-evident. The disease label removes from the individual some of the accompanying sense of guilt. The blame which can be attached is substantially diminished. The removal of the sense of sin as a precondition of altered behaviour is recognised by the church in its stress on forgiveness as the basis for a new life. As a patient, the alcoholic can expect to be excused work as a right and to be spared the full weight of moral condemnation. Unfortunately, the disease label carries the implication that treatment will effect a cure and that the responsibility for cure lies with doctors. In fact the results of treating alcoholics in mental hospitals are generally disappointing. Success depends upon the enthusiasm of follow up after the acute phase is over and involvement of the 'patients' in group work of one sort or another. On the other hand, the removal of guilt and the possibility that the alcoholic can regard himself as suffering from a biochemical abnormality or an 'allergy' which makes it impossible for him to use alcohol, has given Alcoholics Anonymous, and the individual alcoholic, a new base from which to achieve sobriety. Alcoholism is a combination of physical and psychological dependence and the less of the latter the better the prognosis. This can be rephrased by saying that 'cure' depends upon an individual's personality resources rather than upon outside intervention.

Psychiatrists in the UK are by and large mechanistic rather

than analytic in their approach: that is, they tend more often to rely on drugs and to conceive of mental illness as analogous to physical illness than to rely on psychotherapeutic and analytic approaches. The mechanistic approach is based upon a belief, for which there is as yet no convincing evidence, that mental illness and especially schizophrenia and endogenous depression, represent a biochemical abnormality. They are therefore, in a true sense, a manifestation of disease rather than failure to function in society. Such an approach is relatively simple, not very time-consuming and has without doubt restored more quickly to health some who are depressed and enabled some schizophrenics to return to life in the community. Such an approach applied to anxiety or depression which is a response to problems of living is much less successful. Not only does it imply that drugs can solve problems but once somebody has been labelled or stigmatised as mentally ill, it is more difficult for them to accept that they are normal, that learning how to cope with their problems is their responsibility. They tend to perceive themselves as marked out as needing continuous help in order to survive and are tempted to use their 'illness' as a mechanism for running away from reality.

Many psychiatrists have, by maintaining that mental illness is akin to physical illness, tried to diminish the stigmatising effects of admission to mental hospital or of obtaining psychiatric help. In this they have been only partially successful (probably more successful in the USA than here) and for most people an admission to a mental hospital has much greater effect on their image of themselves than admission to an ordinary hospital. The suggestion that somebody needs, or would benefit from, the help of a professional psychiatrist has to be broached with extreme care because for many people this still implies that at worst they are mad or at best that they should become, for the time being at any rate, second class citizens. One of the unfortunate results of this cultural conception, which is often reinforced by doctors who are not themselves psychiatrists, is that students and especially medical students may be very reluctant to seek help with their problems. Student counsellors are important not only because of the help they can give but also because they are not directly associated with psychiatrists.

The problems associated with an analytic approach are somewhat different. The first is logistic: an analysis is very time consuming and it is, unless there were many more analysts, not possible to make it widely available. It is probably impossible to undertake an analysis unless patient and analyst share the same cultural background and usually similar social class. Lastly, evidence that either formal analysis or simpler psychotherapy do good, is both difficult to assess and largely lacking. The advantage of a psychotherapeutic approach is that it does not suggest that the responsibility for solving problems lies with the therapist.

For all these reasons, I made relatively little use of psychiatric colleagues. Most of my referrals were for custodial care: depressed patients judged to be at risk of suicide, manic patients whose behaviour was threatening the economic survival of their families, alcoholics at a crisis. I relatively seldom needed help with diagnosis (psychiatric diagnoses are often a matter of opinion rather than established fact and seldom predict definitive treatment), but occasionally I referred patients to an analyst. The very large number of patients attending psychiatric outpatients represents, in part, the reluctance of many doctors to devote time to listening and sometimes their rejection of patients as difficult, 'bad' or as having 'inadequate personalities'.

Psychiatrists, like other doctors, prefer patients who recover from illness. They have, nonetheless, a responsibility for the long term care of a considerable number of schizophrenics, of the mentally handicapped, of some elderly dements, psychogeriatrics, and a small number of disturbed and violent people. The interface between prison and mental hospital is not sharply defined and prisons not only contain an undue proportion of people with minor degrees of mental handicap but also a number who by ordinary criteria can be judged as psychiatrically sick.[1]

The number of mental hospital beds is much greater than is usually realised as most are provided on separate sites – many of them previously asylums. While the term lunatic asylum has fallen into disfavour, it is a pity that the need to dispense with lunatics as a description has also rid us of the notion of an asylum or refuge. The needs of the mentally handicapped, the demented and many of the mentally ill are much better described as asylum where they can be protected and cared for, a refuge from the problems, cares and demands of the outside world, rather than as a hospital from which they can expect treatment and cure.

Psychiatry is not a popular specialty and like geriatrics finds it difficult to recruit a fair share of talented doctors. Its relatively lowly place in the medical school hierarchy and its rejection by teachers who conceive of illness in mechanistic terms are in part responsible. In addition, and despite protestations to the contrary, mental illness is still not culturally acceptable: it is not viewed as respectable or as being analogous to physical illness. There are of course individual and to some extent social class exceptions to such a sweeping generalisation and the number of people who no longer find the suggestion of seeking psychiatric help unacceptable is growing. Nonetheless, most people are reluctant to admit that either they, or their close relatives, have been in mental hospitals and certainly feel that such knowledge would prejudice them in seeking a job.

Obstetrics

Present obstetric practice has been severely criticised, and not without justification. Pregnancy has been transformed from a normal physiological process into an illness: an illness which demands involvement with doctors and almost always an admission to hospital. This has made a contribution to reducing maternal and perinatal mortality (which mortality includes foetal deaths after the 28th week, stillbirths and deaths in the first week of life). Perinatal mortality is important not only of itself but because its causes are also the causes of mental handicap and measures which reduce mortality will also reduce handicap. This is now widely recognised and has led, particularly in France, to the development of a national policy, involving considerable resource allocation aimed to reduce both perinatal mortality and mental handicap.[2]

It is difficult to disentangle the relative contributions of professional care, improvements in maternal nutrition, and the effects of family planning (in reducing the number of large families and the number of elderly mothers), to improved results. In addition, therapeutic abortion is beginning to have some – although as yet numerically small – effect. Theoretically, the possibility of identifying major defects while the foetus is still *in utero* coupled with the use of therapeutic abortion could substantially reduce the number of infants born with serious handicap.

Pregnancy and labour should – and very often can – be a time of happiness and fulfilment, ending in the birth of a healthy baby. Too often pregnancy is envisaged as a hazardous journey, associated with numerous discomforts and culminating in an agony. Normal labour, and the word is well chosen, is hard work. With the arrogance of those who have never given birth, I believe the experience should be analogous to any hard physical task which has a clear goal. It might be compared to running a mile competitively or climbing a mountain: certainly discomfort is involved, certainly one is making a major effort, but the goal is clearly ascertainable and the discomfort can be readily contained. I am not against the use of drugs for pain relief but they should not be necessary as a routine.

The contrasts between the pregnant woman continuing happily with her ordinary tasks until labour begins and then continuing to walk around, sit or lie down as she feels appropriate in the company of her husband and family, and the dash to the maternity hospital are considerable. On the one hand, as labour advances she has family and friends to talk to, a husband's arm to grasp and the possibility of squatting, the physiological position for delivery.[3] On the other hand, she is put to bed in a strange environment; strangers shave and prepare her; she may be allowed to walk around but her fears and her pains produce tablets and injections rather than love; vaginal and abdominal examinations take place from time to time; she may be confined to bed and attached to a device to monitor the heart beat of the baby. Ultimately she will be delivered in an unphysiological position, sometimes while unconscious, sometimes drugged and sometimes deprived of sensation by an epidural block. This is of course a caricature of modern obstetric care but it is not a total lie.

In as much as it is not a lie it is important for several reasons. It diminishes the woman's autonomy in an important event in her life. It prevents her from sharing the experience with those who love her. It reduces her sense of responsibility for successful delivery. In a way she is no longer allowed to feel that she has had the baby: it was the doctors and the nurses who produced it, not she herself. This has two serious consequences. First, it makes a contribution to perpetuating the view that childbirth is an illness, that having children is a disease. Secondly, it diminishes the chance that the infant will be accepted from the moment of its birth as a wonderful achievement, something to be gathered into one's arms, placed to the breast and loved. Kempe, who first described 'battered babies', now rather dully known as non-accidental injury to children, claims that by observing labour and delivery and noticing to what extent the mother accepts or rejects the infant, he can predict 75 per cent of children who will subsequently be injured.[4] There is a fear that 'bonding failure', failure of the mother to accept and love the infant, may in time allow the baby to develop into a permanently scarred individual who is for ever incapable of making successful relationships. This is more likely if the baby is whisked away as it may well be if its condition is giving rise to concern or if it is born prematurely.

Bourne has drawn attention to the problems which surround a stillbirth.[5] A stillbirth is a tragedy for both mother and the staff who have been caring for her. Sometimes there is the additional problem that the baby is seriously deformed. Faced with this situation, doctors and nurses tend to be at a loss: a funereal silence and long faces characterise the labour ward. The mother is avoided and the remains bundled away, ultimately to be disposed of without the normal rituals of death. The mother is usually denied the possibility of focusing her grief on a real baby, something she has seen, loved even briefly and which was part of her. Instead she is left to mourn something of whose existence there is no proof, something so horrible that she was not allowed to know.

Physiological Birth

There is little new in advocating a restoration of a physiological approach to pregnancy and labour. What is surprising is that so long after Grantly Dick Read and the widespread adoption of relaxation classes and other preparation, labour is still so seldom joyful.

One of the aspects of the modern management of labour that has been severely criticised is the use of induction. Obviously it is good practice to induce labour when to allow it to continue carries an increased risk to the unborn child. Unfortunately, the development of safe methods of inducing labour and the use of intravenous drips containing oxytocic drugs (drugs which stimulate uterine contraction) to control the progress of labour, offered the possibility of planned birth. It was argued that if babies could be born during normal working hours, one could guarantee that all necessary staff would be available to deal with emergencies.

Birth, like death, has become, not one of the incontrovertible facts of life, but something dirty, shameful, fit only for hardened professional eyes. It is difficult not to share the view of those who feel that children should experience both birth and death and that protecting them carries the risk of perpetual immaturity. Efforts have been made to encourage fathers to be present at delivery although it is still the exception rather than the rule. One of the many advantages of having babies at home is that not only husbands but children can share in the experience.

It is probably now impossible to make home delivery usual rather than the diminishing exception. With good antenatal care most problems or potentially dangerous situations can be anticipated and in many instances unforeseen difficulties during labour can be dealt with by transfer to hospital. In Holland where many, although now a diminishing number, of deliveries still take place at home, figures for maternal and perinatal mortality are enviably low. Nonetheless, a return to domiciliary delivery in the UK would imply, as preconditions, a demand to have babies at home, and adequately trained and motivated doctors and midwives. Unless experienced doctors and midwives were available, the inevitable price would be some, probably small, number of unnecessary deaths of mothers and babies.

There were great strengths in the relationship between

family doctor and patient that envisaged a continuity, which stretched from being at the birth of a child to helping that child's children into the world. Over a much shorter span there are great strengths in one doctor's responsibility encompassing family planning, antenatal care, delivery and postnatal care for both mother and baby. The physical aspects of antenatal care are very simple and are mainly concerned with the regular monitoring of very simple things such as weight, blood pressure, uterine size and the presence of foetal movements. They are delegatable in large part to a nurse. The emotional and psychological aspects are not as simple and are often ignored. Those who attend hospital antenatal clinics are likely to see a different junior doctor on each occasion, in an environment which precludes real privacy and in an atmosphere which is inimical to communication. Their physical status will be accurately determined, their emotional needs neither discovered nor satisfied.

A single practitioner who is responsible for the totality of antenatal care has the opportunity to build a relationship of mutual confidence and respect which can be a great asset during labour and which may continue for many years afterwards. The general practitioner unit which allows him to supervise delivery in an institutional setting is a good compromise, especially when it is closely related to a specialist unit. If a general practitioner is to be actively engaged in obstetrics he must be both properly trained and practising his art. Within a practice population of 2,500, depending on its age structure, there will be some 40–50 births a year. The practitioner obstetrician should not be dealing with less: if he is to be present during labour, and at some deliveries, this means a major disruption of ordinary schedules, and is only possible if he is a member of a group practice.

Few present day practitioners or young entrants are prepared to contemplate accepting responsibility for home deliveries and our dwindling corps of midwives is becoming out of practice. Improvement in obstetric care depends upon greater emphasis on emotional and psychological aspects and enabling and encouraging more doctors to become involved. The specialist obstetrician regards the normal delivery as not requiring and as being wasteful of his time and skills: there is still a place for the general practitioner.

14 GENERAL PRACTICE

Competence

For most people in the UK, 'my doctor' refers to a general practitioner. In the United States, where general practice is sparsely distributed, people are more apt to talk about 'my psychiatrist', 'my surgeon', or 'my cardiologist'. In both cultures the use of the possessive 'my' implies something personal about the relationship. It is not uncommon to overhear people defending, in an impassioned way, the virtues of *their* doctors and sometimes categorising the vices of other people's. It is a pity that more doctors do not hear the catalogue of their failings as seen by members of their community: this would be a useful corrective to the fulsome compliments they receive from their admirers.

General practice is characterised by a much greater degree of variability of standards and of approach than hospital practice. The reasons for this are partly historical. Before 1952 the newly qualified could go into practice immediately. Since then an intern year, a year spent as a junior hospital doctor has been necessary before full registration. Even now, although there are proposals and draft legislation to make some postgraduate training mandatory, the newly registered doctor can enter general practice at once and accept unsupervised responsibility for the care of patients.

As a result, most doctors who are in general practice have become general practitioners without any specific training and with a variable, and sometimes limited, experience of post-graduate work in hospital. Quite a number have spent a year as an assistant to a more senior doctor, either with a view to partnership or as a trainee. In either event the emphasis during the year is likely to have been on learning by being thrown in at the deep end, rather than on a carefully and conscientiously supervised apprenticeship.

The choice of general practice as a career was more often dictated by economic necessity than a positive desire to work in the community. Many entered practice because they had no hope of being selected for further training and ultimately a consultant post, or because marriage and other commitments made earning a more realistic livelihood in the immediate future essential. In the fifties and early sixties a number of doctors who had spent many years training for a specialty ultimately became time-expired registrars and reluctantly decided to enter practice.

In all these instances those who became practitioners either from choice or necessity entered practice in total ignorance of the real nature of the work that they were expected to do. Their previous training had been confined to the laboratory and the hospital, especially the teaching hospital. In the novel situation in which they found themselves their past experience was of a very limited value.

Many of the patients that they saw had complaints which could not be fitted into neat diagnostic categories. Used to diagnostic certainty they were faced with uncertainty and often lacked a senior colleague to whom they could turn for advice. Furthermore they were now the decision makers and patients expected their doctors to manage, as a rule, without recourse to a second opinion. Access to investigations was difficult and could not be used as a device to postpone a decision. Somewhat to their surprise most of their patients accepted the proffered diagnosis and treatment and most of them recovered and were duly grateful. Gradually they developed, as a result of experience, assurance. As the experience was acquired in isolation and not submitted to critical examination, it allowed them to continue to make the same mistakes with increasing confidence. They knew, as a result of experience, that examining patients seldom affected the response to treatment: they knew that injections of vitamins were good for tiredness and they knew that flu was an acceptable diagnosis.

They quickly came to realise that general practice was different from hospital medicine and even if their erstwhile colleagues were critical and sometimes scathing about the competence of general practitioners, it didn't really matter; they were making a livelihood and their patients loved them.

In the early 1950s a group of general practitioners, under the guidance of John Hunt, now Lord Hunt, founded an academic College of General Practitioners. This marked a turning point. It was an effort, though not the first, to recognise general practice as a discipline in its own right rather than the practice of hospital medicine in a community setting.[1] Twenty-five years later only about 30 per cent of practitioners are associated with this College as Members or Fellows, and many doctors find its activities pretentious or irrelevant and see membership as a means of seeking self-advancement.

Objective evidence of variability derives from an examination of the equipment and environment in which doctors work. It has been shown that many practitioners lack what most would consider basic tools, and that some surgeries and waiting rooms are a disgrace.[2] A visit to an out-patient department of a major hospital will still provide ample evidence of a low standard of competence in general practice. Not only are many referral letters inadequate but it is not difficult to point to major errors of omission and commission. Fortunately, low standards of competence are probably associated with high referral rates. Doctors who record their referral rates tend to be competent so that this observation is conjecture rather than fact. The examination for Membership of the Royal College of General Practitioners (MRCGP) shows that most domestic graduates who choose to present themselves are satisfactory according to the criteria used: it can tell us nothing about those who do not wish to be examined.

The high and even level of competence in hospital has been achieved by protracted specialist training, competition for posts and peer review. In the past none of these conditions was satisfied in general practice and the inevitable result was variation in the quality of care.

Overseas doctors have been employed in very considerable

numbers to provide the junior hospital staff thought to be necessary to run our hospitals. Many of them do not aspire to a career in this country, but those who do tend to be driven into unpopular specialties where they are not competing with domestic graduates. As a result, an undue proportion find consultant employment as geriatricians and psychiatrists and a number work as principals in practice, mostly in unpopular and under-doctored areas. The examination for the MRCGP has shown that some of these doctors lack knowledge which we would expect of graduates. This reflects not on their ability, but on the nature of their undergraduate training. It is a cause of concern because it may be that a minimum essential standard is not always being maintained. The overseas doctor is also at a disadvantage unless he is working within a familiar culture. The Englishman in India, or the Indian in Britain may occasionally carry a special aura of ability to heal, but both are at a disadvantage in trying to provide primary care – especially in psychological and social terms – in an alien culture. This is also true of psychiatry but relatively unimportant in surgery.

This account focuses on the shortcomings and failings of general practice. On the credit side practitioners have provided an open access service to the whole population, and provided it immediately. On the whole they achieved remarkably good relationships with the vast majority of patients, they immunised a high proportion of the public, introduced preventive procedures for the first time in any curative medical service. A few made outstanding contributions to our knowledge.

Workload

Despite variability, almost all practices seem to have a workload problem, which is manifest as the six-minute consultation. This is sometimes difficult to understand when examining published figures.

There is evidence that the number of consultations/per patient/per year has been falling steadily, although there is still a wide variation. This could be due to greater use of nurses and other non-doctor personnel. It could be due to a change in the nature of disease in the community or to a change in patients' perceptions of what it was useful to bring to doctors. It is probably determined in large part by doctors themselves. Not only do they decide if and when a patient should return; they can also discourage patients from attending with certain sorts of problems. In this way they have a major influence in determining their work. How they behave will be related to how they are paid. It has been suggested that, given supporting staff, doctors in the NHS could provide high quality care for many more people than at present. Certainly doctors in other places, especially parts of Scandinavia, appear to do so successfully. Unfortunately, available measures of high quality care are largely lacking. Judged by crude statistics which measure mortality this statement stands. It may be true if the general practitioner is to confine his activity to the management of physical symptoms and the diagnosis of serious physical disease. If he is, in addition, to provide emotional support, counselling and psychotherapy, and to play a full part in the prevention of disease, his ability to care for more than 2,500 patients, even when he is provided with staff, must be open to question.

The amount of time allotted to surgery consultations is usually determined by tradition within the practice rather than being the result of any form of work study. If the expectation of patients and the pattern of practice of doctors is a brief consultation, then it is easy to predict that only sufficient time to achieve this will be allowed. One of the mechanisms doctors use to maintain the necessary momentum in the surgery and an adequately speedy turnover is a full waiting room. The existence of so many awaiting their turn deters the individual patient from seeking to protract the consultation. Furthermore, the doctor can successfully point out, sometimes in non-verbal ways, how busy he is, how real are the pressures under which he has to work. The popular stereotype of the general practitioner always includes the notion that he is busy, and doctors capitalise on this and make a substantial contribution to the maintenance of something that is, in part, a myth.

A number of highly organised and well motivated doctors now arrange special clinics, for antenatal care for example and many have an arrangement which allows for relatively lengthy appointments for special purposes such as psychotherapy or counselling.

Good practice is only possible when time is properly controlled and used. Although the intrusion of emergencies and unexpected demands cause occasional havoc to ordered plans, this is not sufficiently frequent to be a major difficulty, although it is always hard to bear. The argument so often heard that something is impossible for lack of time is more often a rationalisation of unwillingness than a statement of fact.

Organisation

Among the most striking changes in general practice since the war has been the growth of partnerships and groups and the increased number of purpose-built premises and health centres. This has been accompanied by a large increase in the numbers of other staff employed by, or working with, doctors and the emergence of what is fashionably known as a team approach.

The single-handed practitioner, still the rule rather than the exception in Ireland, provided a twenty-four hour service for 365 days a year. It was difficult, in past times, when competition for patients existed, for the doctor to have a holiday or time off for relaxation, and it almost precluded attendance at refresher courses or other forms of postgraduate training. Such a doctor, motivated in part by economic pressures, provided real continuity of care and normally responded to all out-of-hours demands. The main disadvantages stemmed from his professional isolation and, if he was busy and had a large practice, from the effects on his family and on the quality of his life. Sometimes in these circumstances middle age was accompanied by a sense of disillusion, a profound weariness which led in its turn to falling standards.

Professional isolation is not confined to the single-handed: it stems more from an attitude of mind than from environment, and many doctors in group practice effectively isolate themselves from the opportunities of learning from their colleagues. Learning requires the conscious creation of opportunities to examine what is being done and to meet in a semi-formal way with other partners or associates.

The increased economic security and the diminution in competition for patients which followed the creation of the National Health Service opened the way to the creation of groups and partnerships. This has steadily continued and single-handed doctors are now the exception. Some of the groups are large and include as many as ten or even more doctors.

Even two doctors working together, or an arrangement to provide off-duty or holiday cover, goes a long way towards eliminating the main disadvantages of single-handed practice. Patients are very ready to recognise the reasonable needs of doctors for time off and respond favourably to the suggestion that doctors need time away from the practice for further study.[3] They recognise that in a small group it is possible to know each of the partners, and believe, sometimes without good reason, that the quality of records provides a link between their own doctor and his colleagues. It is said, and this is sometimes justified, that allegiance has been transferred from the individual doctor to the group. It is easy to maintain that this may be possible in a group of three or four doctors, but it becomes a nonsense if the group consists of ten.

While people recognise the need for doctors to have tim off and are reasonably happy under these circumstances t see a partner rather than their own doctor, they have becom very resentful about the extent to which out-of-hours care i now provided by strange doctors or by deputising services This is seen as unreasonable and in direct conflict with thei expectation of a personal relationship with their doctor, an a commitment by him to them as individuals.

Another recent change in general practice has been th emphasis on organisation and the close involvement of other not only secretaries and receptionists but also nurses, healt visitors and social workers. Appointment systems are no much more widely used. While ostensibly these are for th convenience of patients they can acquire as their main pu pose the protection of doctors. For those who possess tel phones the ability to make an appointment and, if fortuna see the doctor without a protracted wait and at a convenie time is a great asset. For those who are elderly or who do not have access to a phone, having to make an appointment can be a powerful deterrent or at least a nuisance. Particular problems arise in the case of those who are seeking an urgent appointment. If the list is already full, the receptionist is placed in an invidious position. If she overbooks, she incurs the wrath of the doctor. If she fails to divert the patient to another partner or successfully discourages or dissuades the patient from being seen that day, she runs the risk of prejudicing health. Predictably those patients whose needs are the greatest are least likely to get their way. Good receptionists who are beloved, whose patience is boundless and whose equanimity cannot be disturbed, are beyond price. Doctors who are so blessed should protect their staff and accept their judgement. They should realise that it is their staff, rather than they themselves, who bear the main brunt of criticism and complaint – most of which should more properly be laid at the doctor's door.

In theory a team approach to problems offers the possibility of better care. In practice it has the danger, eloquently put by Sir Theodore Fox, that 'the particular object of his [the doctor's] independent existence may be defeated if he leaves all dressings to the nurse, sympathy to the receptionist, messages to the secretary and the solution of home problems to the social worker . . . If somebody else is to do all the small things for the patient under the doctor's distant supervision, personal contact will be reduced to a minimum . . .'[4] It may result in a dilution of ultimate responsibility and a failure to grasp the realities of the situation. Activity, and referral from person to person, may become a substitute for tackling the core of the problem.

The Large City

Certain environments create special problems. The most important of these, because it affects so many people, is the large city. Characteristically, few people now live at the centre of large cities. The immediate centre is surrounded by a densely populated but impoverished area. Further out, housing estates and corporation flats appear and even further removed are the areas inhabited by the affluent and the upper middle class. The city centre tends to have two populations and two lives: a daytime population of people working or shopping and a night-time population seeking entertainment and diversion. The night-time population can be further divided into the respectable, seeking theatres and restaurants, and the deprived seeking stimulus and excitement.

Doctors who belong, regardless of their origins, to the middle class, almost never choose to live in, or to be identified with, a community which is exclusively working class or an area which is undesirable. As a result, not only are such areas underdoctored but an undue proportion of their doctors work there not by choice, but 'faute de mieux'. Tudor Hart's Inverse Care Law which states that where the need for services is greatest the services are poorest, applies.[5] Few of the doctors live in the community they serve, they do not identify with it and they confine themselves to working there during the daytime from what, in the past, was deprecatingly referred to as a 'lock-up surgery', which was often nothing more than a converted shop and provided minimal facilities. Such a generalisation is not invalidated by the occasional exception.

Those who live in the depressed areas near to the centre of cities have many disadvantages. There is an undue proportion of immigrants, social problems are commonplace, insecurity and high mobility usual. Some areas develop a sense of community based upon shared ethnic origin and a few original urban communities have survived rehousing schemes. Adjoining the most deprived areas is 'bed-sitter land', most obvious in London and predominantly female.

Two other characteristics of large cities are worth mentioning: one is the existence of large hospitals near the city centre, the other is the population of single homeless, sleeping rough, using hostels, many of whom are alcoholics and some of whom are 'schizophrenes'.

General practice fails to provide an adequate service for those who live near to the heart of large towns. There is, however, an alternative source of primary – that is, direct access – medical care, the accident and emergency or casualty department. These departments deal with the accidents and acute misfortunes of those who temporarily inhabit the city centre. On the whole, despite the relatively junior standing of most of the doctors, this task is well done. They are at their best in dealing with emergencies which are physical rather than emotional: this is what they have been trained to manage.

Sparsely populated areas also have special problems, but their nature is different. As a general rule people who live in isolated places are self-reliant and have a low demand for care. This may reflect the difficulty of reaching doctors but probably also reflects a philosophy which accepts minor degrees of discomfort as inevitable. Many are self-employed and small farmers are reluctant to become sick because of the ensuing problems: cows demand to be milked, stock has to be watered. In the United Kingdom, where such areas are few and the number of doctors relatively large, there has been little difficulty in recruiting doctors to work in out-of-the-way places. These doctors tend to share some of the characteristics of their patients and enjoy isolation and the challenge of having to rely on their own resources.

The GP in Hospital

Many general practitioners do other jobs part time – most commonly, clinical assistantships in hospital. They also work as factory doctors, police surgeons and school medical officers. A number now hold part-time posts in education, particularly in connection with postgraduate training for general practice but also in university departments.

There has been renewed interest in the role of small local or cottage hospitals staffed by practitioners. There are many more of these than is generally realised and they play an important part in the life of their communities. Such hospitals, by providing nursing care in an institutional setting, allow practitioners to look after patients (who would otherwise have to be admitted to general hospitals) near to their homes and to their relations. In addition they can accept patients for convalescence from other hospitals at an early stage, thus reducing pressure on beds. They also have a potential place in the care of the dying. The danger is that all their beds become occupied by long-stay elderly patients and if this is allowed to happen their usefulness may be diminished.

Training for General Practice

It was long recognised that practitioners, particularly those working alone, needed refresher courses so as to keep their knowledge up to date. More recently, doctors have been bribed to attend by making seniority payments conditional on attendance at recognised courses. In Ireland doctors in the General Medical Services Scheme have been paid a lump sum each year to enable them to take time off for educational purposes. In practice the good effects of these efforts have been diminished by the nature of the teaching, which has, in general, been didactic. The usual format is a lecture by a specialist on some aspect of his specialty. As a result teaching has sometimes been irrelevant and learning minimal. Nonetheless, the development of Postgraduate Medical Centres and the appointment of tutors to organise courses has improved the previous state of affairs.

Drug companies have also played a part, not only in promoting their products, but also by generous sponsorship of educational activities organised by others. Those doctors who are least in need of continuing education are predictably the most assiduous in its pursuit. The habit of reading major periodicals has to be acquired early, ideally while still a student. Although the most widely read are the 'give away' newspapers and periodicals sponsored directly or indirectly by drug houses, every member of the British Medical Association and every member of the College of General Practitioners receive their journals. Other methods of self-instruction particularly tape/slide presentations, pioneered by John and Valerie Graves as the Medical Recording Service of the Royal College of General Practitioners, have grown steadily in popularity.

The fundamental problem is not the provision of courses or the circulation of periodicals or other reading matter; the problem is ensuring that doctors themselves recognise the need for lifelong learning as normal and essential. In fairness there is no other profession which has taken the task of continuing education so seriously. In America and Canada the question of recertification has been seriously debated and many doctors in the USA are now undergoing formal reassess ment of their knowledge and competence.

The influence of drug houses has been severely criticised and recently the British government has tried to control promotional expenditure. In addition to meetings, accompanied by excellent food and drink, vast amounts of advertising material arrive daily through the post. Samples and gimmicks, calendars, biros, even sphygmomanometers are given away. Representatives call on a regular basis and local chemists aver that they can tell who has recently been in the district by alterations in prescribing.

The most significant change in general practice in the last fifteen years has been the gradual acceptance that even if it is not a specialty in its own right, which many believe, doctors who are going to make it their career require special postgraduate training. The full effects of making vocational training (postgraduate in-service training in a specialty) mandatory will not be felt until many, or the majority of doctors in practice, have undergone such training. That will take many years. Nonetheless, the acceptance in principle, which is likely to be extended throughout the European Community, has had a number of healthy immediate effects.

Already there are almost 1,500 young men and women enrolled in courses of training for general practice in the UK. As a rule they spend two years (sometimes eighteen months) in hospital, and a year in supervised practice. During their hospital posts they attend other teaching programmes on a day release basis. As a result, a large number of practitioners have had to become teachers, have learned to examine what they do in a critical way and have, as a result, improved their own practice.

The Future

General practice as we know it – a primary health care service directly accessible on demand and based upon doctors – is a luxury. It is a luxury that only wealthy nations can afford. In a world context there are few countries who have sufficient doctors in relation to population to deploy them in this way. Increasingly, poorer countries are providing a community service based upon local people who have had a relatively brief training which has concentrated upon prevention rather than cure. The most widely known of these is the Chinese 'barefoot doctor'.

One extreme view, held by those whose experience of general practice is generally secondhand, sees the role of the practitioner as nothing more than a buffer between an insatiable demand for care and the hospital service. By sorting the serious from the trivial, general practitioners prevent the hospitals being swamped. Otherwise they do little more than issue certificates, usually for inadequate reasons, and indulge in a variable amount of hand holding depending on their nature and inclinations. At the other extreme some doctors, mostly general practitioners, conscious of the extent of specialisation within hospital (few consultant posts are now advertised for general physicians without the addition of a specified special interest), see the general practitioner as the general physician of the future: a doctor who, because of his training in internal medicine, is competent to manage the majority of medical conditions and who will use his specialist colleagues as and when he deems it necessary. They see the practitioner as conducting an orchestra of professional skills in the interests of a patient with whom he has a continuing relationship and whom he knows.

Some would see general practice as nothing more than the use of hospital skills in a different setting; others would maintain its right to be considered a separate and unique academic discipline. Is the general practitioner a 'Jack of all trades and master of none', or can he aspire to be a master in a field of his own? Despite the Royal College and despite academic departments, many doctors remain unconvinced of general practice's right to be considered a separate discipline.

The critical question which remains concerns the cost benefit of providing a primary health care service staffed by doctors. Determining cost benefit demands an examination of the nature of the inputs, the cost and nature of the process, and the outcomes. The inputs are determined by society's conception of the doctor's role. At the moment doctors seldom reach out into the 'healthy' community to create work, and their work is initially determined by the patient's decision to consult. The subsequent course of events, the number of repeat consultations, is largely determined by the doctor, varies with workload, and is affected by the way in which he is paid. A different society which did not regard doctors as making any contribution to solving problems of living, or a society which did not require certification of illness would generate different and possibly lesser demands upon its doctors. If nurses were to replace doctors as the professionals to whom people had direct access, and if doctors could be seen only by referral, it is possible that the problems with which doctors would have to deal would be different. Such a change might, however, be seen as a reduction in the quality of the service and be fiercely resisted. If it were pushed through against opposition, it could lead to the emergence, or recrudescence, of private general practice. In the short term the possibility of replacing or eliminating general practice is, in the UK, entirely hypothetical; although it is certainly conceivable that some alternative way of providing care may be developed in large cities.

Within general practice, the process that occurs after the consultation has been initiated has already been described. The costs derive from doctors' and other staff salaries, the cost and maintenance of premises and the cost of drugs. It has been assumed that the increase in non-medical staff has been beneficial and worthwhile. It is easy to demonstrate that such staff are busy and that they can diminish the doctor's workload. It is difficult to demonstrate that they have reduced mortality or morbidity or even that they have improved the quality of life.

For those who are responsible for decisions regarding expenditure – and in a sense this includes each one of us voting citizens – the major difficulty is the measurement of outcomes, of end results: what difference does it make? What is the real difference between good and bad general practice? Does a shiny health centre make a contribution to the health or happiness of the community it serves? It may be a nice place in which to wait, a showpiece for visitors, or comfortable to work in. Do these considerations alone justify the cost?

Lacking answers to these questions – and surely we must seek, despite the difficulties, proper answers – it may be said with confidence that good general practice is distinguishable from bad. Good general practice is not necessarily more expensive; it may be marginally cheaper. A decision to persist with a health service which includes general practice is, at the moment, reasonable. It may be a luxury: it is one that we can probably afford.

15 THE DOCTOR AND SOCIETY

Public Health

So far the main concern and emphasis in this book has been the role of the doctor in relation to the individual. The centre-piece has been the doctor/patient relationship, the relationship between an individual doctor and an individual patient. Doctors also play a part, sometimes devote a career, as in the case of doctors in the public health service, to the development and provision of services, not to individuals, but to communities and to society as a whole.

Those who devote a career to these aspects are to be found in the public health service as community physicians, and in departments of health. The community physician is the present-day descendant of the Medical Officer of Health. As a group, community physicians are characterised by low status in the eyes of both the profession and society at large, and generally – certainly until recently – relatively low income. They have considerable difficulty in attracting young men and women of calibre to their ranks.

This is unjust because the contribution of doctors in the public service to improvements in the health of our society has been at least as great, if not greater, than the contributions of physicians and surgeons. The control of infectious disease, clean food, air and water, improved sanitation and to a lesser extent housing, have created, even in large cities, a remarkably healthy environment very different from that which obtained one hundred years ago. Their present-day role is somewhat different as the necessary monitoring services, carried out by public health inspectors and reinforced by legislation, have a momentum of their own which now requires only distant supervision.

The reason for their low status and income and their recruitment difficulties is in part due to the self-image of those who take up medicine as a career; partly due to the orientations of present-day medical education, and also in part due to society's lack of familiarity with the work they do and its importance. Few people who aspire to become doctors see their job as the prevention of disease or the administration of health services. Their preoccupations are with serving suffering humanity in a very direct way by curing their diseases. Generally speaking those specialties which do not involve direct involvement with individual patients are relatively unpopular and do not attract many undergraduates. This includes not only the public health service and community health, but also radiology, other laboratory disciplines and basic sciences allied to medicine, such as physiology and anatomy.

The objective of the undergraduate curriculum is no longer the production of a safe general practitioner, but since the Todd report, the qualification of a doctor capable of pursuing further training in his chosen discipline. Medical education has yet to accept and adapt to this change of emphasis.[1] Despite the introduction of behavioural science, sociology and departments of social medicine or community health, the emphasis in medical schools is still upon the treatment of the individual patient. Those who try to stress the importance of prevention, of involvement in the provision of health services, have to struggle not only with unwilling students, but also with colleagues who do not accept its importance.

The scientific discipline associated with public health is epidemiology. Its boundaries have been extended from the study of epidemic disease to include the study of the distribution of diseases and the examination and monitoring of health services. The distribution of disease includes the characterisation of those who contract the disease, their age sex and social class and the seasonal and geographical variation. This approach has added considerably to our knowledge of the cause of disease and has pointed the way to methods of prevention even when the mechanisms of causation have not been understood. John Snow, by studying the distribution of cases of cholera in London in 1853, was able to show that most of them were associated with a particular water supply. Although the organism concerned had not been discovered and knowledge of the importance of preventing faecal contamination of water supplies was lacking, he controlled the outbreak by removing the handle of the Broad Street Pump.

More recently, epidemiological approaches have provided a great deal of evidence for the part played by environmental factors in the aetiology of cancers and have led to appropriate preventive measures especially in industry. The exact cause of premature mortality from coronary heart disease remains unknown but nonetheless epidemiology has identified the characteristics of those most likely to be affected and can point the way to prevention.

Epidemiology, whether concerned with the study of specific diseases or with the provision of health services, relies on the careful accumulation of data, its analysis and interpretation. Little if any of this requires a traditional medical qualification and more and more epidemiologists, statisticians and computer experts are working in the field without having a medical degree. But as yet there is no head of an academic department in these islands who lacks one. Medical knowledge is an advantage to an epidemiologist but he only requires a medical qualification to enhance his status.

In addition to responsibility for environmental control the Medical Officer of Health had traditional responsibilities for the control of infectious disease and for preventive services in general. As environmental control became routine and infectious diseases less important, preventive services, especially the routine examination of children, expanded to become a major activity. It had the advantage that it allowed doctors working in the public health service to exercise clinical skills, to operate in an area where their medical training seemed relevant. Since this time, the value of examining school children in a routine way has been seriously questioned and the emphasis has shifted to developmental assessment – that is, the examination of infants and toddlers. A mystique has grown around developmental paediatrics, and while the techniques used to detect minor degrees of abnormality, especially of the nervous system and special senses, require learning, it sometimes seems that their difficulty has been exaggerated. The Court Report, while recognising that many doctors in the public health service will continue for the time being to be involved in child care, recommends that in the future most preventive services should be provided by general practitioners.[2]

Particularly since the reorganisation of the National Health Service in 1974, the descendants of Medical Officers of Health, district community physicians, their staff, area and regional medical officers, have had to survive considerable changes, sometimes involving moving to a new area and they are still uncertain of their role. The title community physician suggests a doctor who diagnoses, treats and ameliorates or cures the problems of a community rather than the ills of an individual. This is probably as good a succinct statement of the task which they are supposed to fulfil as any other. Diagnosis rests on accumulating the necessary facts, and data collection and information services are seen as being increasingly important. The advantages of being a doctor in this situation are of two sorts; advantages which derive from knowledge and advantages which derive from status. The newly fledged graduate certainly lacks the necessary training as a specialist in community medicine which emphasises epidemiology, demography, sociology and statistics. This training is protracted and is designed not only to provide the necessary knowledge and skills but also to establish community medicine as a recognised specialty and to ensure that such specialists will be entitled to the same rates of pay as their hospital colleagues. The theoretical advantage of doctor status is that it enhances the possibility that the community physician will obtain the co-operation of, and be able to influence, professional colleagues. In practice this advantage has been diminished by the low status accorded to the specialty. Doctors in the public health service are seen as second-class doctors, as not being 'real' doctors, as being administrators and bureaucrats. As always, a specialty which is poorly staffed, underpaid and out of the mainstream of medical education, tends like the poor to remain poor and to grow poorer, while the already rich grow richer.

Academic departments of social medicine and the recently established Faculty of Community Medicine in the Royal College of Physicians of London have begun to redress the balance. The main strength of university departments has been in epidemiology, which is now respectable, and many of them are becoming involved in health service planning and operational research. While this is welcome and helps to restore the balance, it has sometimes seemed to divide academic and practical community medicine and run the danger of further isolating those doctors in the public health service.

The community physician of the future will require administrative skills and should function as an epidemiologist, be able to collect useful data, be expert in its analysis and proficient in monitoring services. Whether such a task is primarily or essentially for doctors must remain an open question.

Doctors, relatively few in number, who work in the Department of Health and Social Security and in the regional departments tend to maintain the anonymity characteristic of career civil servants. It is, therefore, difficult to assess their contribution. The rest of the profession tends to be ambivalent in its attitude towards them and sometimes acts as if they had joined the other side. This is an ambivalence which extends to the Department itself, which is often, and frequently unfairly, seen as an unresponsive bureaucracy incapable of decision making. My own, inevitably limited, contacts with these doctors would suggest that they, by virtue of their medical qualification, bring not only expertise to the Department but make a contribution to bridging the gap which exists between it and the profession. Chief Medical Officers wield considerable influence and recent holders of the office, such as Sir George Godber, have used that power constructively and imaginatively.

Many other doctors have only a minimal direct involvement with patients. This is particularly true of those who staff the laboratories and x-ray departments of hospitals, those who work in basic science departments and in the pharmacological industry. The numbers involved are very considerable and it is important that those who insist that an interest and liking for human beings should be a criterion for entry to medicine, recognise that many doctors spend their lives in the laboratory rather than at the bedside.

Generally speaking such doctors are accorded lesser status and have lower incomes than surgeons and physicians. Recruitment of medically qualified staff is difficult, especially in basic science departments such as anatomy and physiology, and more and more people without medical qualifications are holding senior posts.

Occupational Health

Occupational health is concerned with workers and their environment. It is in some sense an offshoot of the public health service and shares its concern with environmental control. Doctors in this field are responsible for ensuring that the health of workers does not suffer as a consequence of their employment. In achieving this aim they have to relate to both workers and management. Trade unions are concerned primarily about the health of their members, management is primarily concerned with the maintenance of a profitable enterprise but usually recognises that the maintenance of the health of workers is ultimately in its best interest.

Generally speaking, doctors in occupational health are not concerned with workers as individuals, although they may examine them to determine their suitability for employment and may re-examine them in a routine way to detect early signs of adverse effects. They may have responsibility for providing a first aid service in the factory but do not ordinarily attempt to supplant the general practitioner in caring for episodic disease.

Examining to determine fitness for work is usually a fairly casual routine designed to protect management at least as much as the worker. There are however some notable exceptions, the most important being those who are going to drive buses, trains, and particularly aeroplanes. Commercial pilots are subjected to intensive examination at regular intervals in order to determine their continued fitness to fly.

The main task of doctors in occupational health is the protection of workers from risk. In this they are aided by legislation and, if they are fortunate and skilful, by co-operative management. Accidents are important and the doctor must ensure, by being thoroughly familiar with conditions on the shop floor, that machinery is protected and most important of all that safety regulations are observed. Many things which contribute to safety, even simple things such as wearing helmets on construction sites, are irksome: unless foremen insist upon compliance, rules will be more honoured in the breach than in the observance. The doctor should understand the place of chemicals and other toxic substances which are used. These can cause harm not only by direct contact but also by inhalation. The ill effects of prolonged exposure to noise have only recently been recognised and in many industries, unless ear plugs or ear muffs are used, many will become permanently deaf.

Some of the unfortunate results of the work environment are not immediately apparent and not only deafness but industrial cancers may take years to develop. For this reason regular monitoring of the health of employees and the notification of illnesses become very important, particularly in order to identify new hazards at the earliest possible moment.

A doctor working in occupational health will be concerned not only with the physical environment but also with general conditions in the factory, with morale and with sickness absence. He should be in a position to advise about the need for adequate breaks, facilities for rest and relaxation, and arrangements which would reduce the tedium of repetitive tasks.

Many of those who are at the moment working in occupational health are part-timers, mostly general practitioners but as the complexity of the specialty grows most large organisations now employ whole time medical staff.

A small number of doctors exert considerable influence through international agencies, most notably the World Health Organisation. The European Community also has a concern with health, and to an increasing extent supranational organisations are influencing health services. This is achieved partly through research and partly through panels of experts who are summoned and invited to make authoritative statements.

Not all doctors are directly involved with patients and many of those who work in the public health service, in government departments and in international organisations, may have a much greater influence on our health than the local practitioner and the neighbourhood hospital.

Allocation of Resource

The major political influence of doctors has been exercised indirectly in that they have determined the directions of health service development on the grounds of special knowledge. It was accepted that they must know best, and civil servants, ministers and governments allowed themselves to be guided by expert advice. The expert advice usually derived from the most prestigious and highly specialised doctors and was a major contributory factor in perpetuating imbalances in health services.

Economic recession has made the selection of priorities and the exercise of choice a necessity. Until fairly recently it was tacitly assumed that in some strange way resources were infinite, and that while all the new hospitals could not be built this year, they would be built next year or the year after. Health services are now a massive industry characterised by a labour-intensive structure. Except insomuch that an efficient service speedily rehabilitates and returns productive workers to their job, it makes no contribution to Gross National Product. It is a non-productive industry and increasing capitalisation, for example new machines and high technology, has not diminished but has tended to increase the work force.

In a situation in which inputs, process and outcomes are controlled, it is possible to arrive at the cost-benefit of modifications and alterations, and relatively easy to make choices. Despite the best efforts of economists and those undertaking operational research, we still lack the tools and the information on which to base rational decisions. The expenditure on attempting this task is, by comparison with total spending in the health service, extremely small. Paradoxically, at a time when such analyses are most needed it is most difficult to create the necessary resource. Many of the choices are in the true sense political and in a democratic society should not be entrusted to doctors or to any other body of experts. Is it more important to improve the quality of life for old people, or to prolong the life of somebody with irreversibly damaged kidneys? Is it more important to buy a CAT scanner or to build a residential home for the mentally handicapped?

The proper grounds for making choices are still elusive. As a general rule our society (including our doctors) favours the acute rather than the chronic, the life threatening rather than the trivial, the curable rather than the incurable, high technology rather than additional staff. At the moment doctors, particularly those who work in outdated hospitals and who see technology as an essential part of progress in care, are unhappy. Simultaneously, their incomes are shrinking, their environment is deteriorating, the prospect of additional resource is lacking and their power to influence the future has apparently disappeared. This has certainly contributed to the recent 'brain drain' of doctors. The decision of the American and Canadian governments to restrict the immigration of doctors may halt this loss but one consequence may be a larger population of dissatisfied doctors.

Proper mechanisms for decision-making regarding the allocation of resource are lacking. The possibilities of inducing change in an industry which is labour intensive at a time of inflation are not great. The breathing space could and should be used to improve the quality of the information which would allow national decision-making acceptable to doctors, politicians and society as a whole.

This utopian situation is still far away and perhaps will remain for ever beyond our reach. In the meantime, the debate about major philosophical questions, the desirable general directions of development and major priorities should be extended beyond the confines of the profession, departments of health or parliaments. This book is a contribution to that wider debate.

Political Power

Relatively few doctors, particularly by comparison with lawyers, have entered political life and few have achieved political eminence. Nonetheless, doctors have been a successful pressure group and have wielded considerable power. They have chosen to confine the exercise of this power to matters of health and have eschewed involvement in broader or more general issues. As a group, their position has always been and still is to the right of centre, and left wing doctors, although they exist, are relatively unusual. Their public image is conservative and the widely publicised attitude of the American Medical Association to the introduction of Medicare and Medicaid may have reinforced this view. Such a view does not do justice to the many doctors, particularly in the public health service, who have been pioneers in social reform. It is often forgotten that the British Medical Association supported the introduction of the National Health Service. This has been overshadowed by their differences of opinion with Aneurin Bevan.

James Murray, Director of the Social Services Council in Ireland, in talking to my students about doctors, referred to the 'overspill of competence into areas in which they possess none. If they were only mechanics, their power would not matter'. I am not sure how important this is but certainly statements made by doctors tend to carry a weight which is ill deserved, particularly when the subject is nothing to do with medicine.

This power may be exercised by the doctor assuming community leadership, particularly in smaller rural communities. It is not necessarily a power for evil and it is at least arguable that doctors, as a group, do not play a sufficiently active part in the communities where they live. The danger lies in what Murray has described as 'the overspill' into matters in which they have no special competence. Such overspill is a feature of our society and not only doctors, but actors, pop stars and footballers, may be invited to pronounce on issues of general interest. Their opinions, particularly when they appear on the printed page, carry considerable, if possibly diminishing, weight.

Much of the doctor's organised power has been exercised through professional organisations. The British Medical Association in many respects acts as the doctor's trade union. In Ireland in addition to the Irish Medical Association there is another organisation, the Medical Union, which is recognised in law. Most, but by no means all, doctors are members of these associations which negotiate salary scales and increases with government. They also from time to time claim to speak for the profession and as they represent not only hospital specialists but also general practitioners, non-consultant doctors and those who work in the public service, this claim is at least partly justified. In common with most large democratic organisations they sometimes seem to be governed by their lowest common denominator and have seldom been in the van in instituting change.

The Royal Colleges, many of whose charters were granted as long ago as the 17th century, are mainly concerned with academic matters and do not usually compete with or intrude upon matters which are the responsibility of the associations. In the past they were concerned with undergraduate education but now, with the sole exception of the Royal College of Surgeons in Ireland, they are predominantly involved in postgraduate training. They have successfully established their examinations as almost a sine qua non for appointment to consultant posts, and have more recently laid down programmes of higher training, which are protracted and out of step with other members of the EEC. There can be no argument that their stranglehold on assessment and training has raised standards; but the strength of their grip has inevitably produced some rigidity and may have enforced over-lengthy periods of apprenticeship.

The governance of the Royal Colleges has usually been in the hands of very senior members of the profession and most Presidents have been near to retiring age. In the London College of Physicians membership, obtained by examination relatively early in a doctor's career, until recently, by no means inevitably led to election to fellowship. Generally speaking the Colleges are now recognising the importance of involving younger men and are beginning to play a more notable public role. A good example is the initiatives taken by the Royal College of Physicians regarding smoking.

The almost bewildering number of colleges, their grades of licentiate, member and fellow, produce a hideous proliferation of letters after doctors' names, which are the despair of our American colleagues, and mean little to anyone except to the members of the doctor's club. There are three Royal Colleges of Physicians, three of Surgeons, and one of Physicians and Surgeons: each of these has faculties, some in anaesthesia, some in radiology, some in community medicine. There are relatively junior colleges now possessing royal charters; they are obstetricians and gynaecologists, general practitioners, pathologists, psychiatrists and radiologists. Each new College aspires to make its membership more difficult and to enhance the standing of the specialty it represents. They acquire silver, chains of office, maces and academic gowns and are ripe for detailed sociological study.

Doctors also exercise power through universities and medical schools. As a general rule medical schools are thought to add to the prestige of universities although their links with the wider university may sometimes appear tenuous. There is a danger that medicine may lose its right to be considered a university discipline if it neglects its roots and becomes even more obviously a technical training. Already doctors have been shown to be narrow, authoritarian, rigid and humourless by comparison with their social science contemporaries.[3]

Perhaps the real need is a return to an earlier tradition which linked medicine to philosophy and the humanities in general. If the proper study of mankind is man, no profession has a greater need to undertake this study. The novel, poetry and history may have an equally important part to play in producing civilised doctors.

16 RESEARCH AND EDUCATION

Research

The idea that research should be a usual or normal part of the doctor's role is relatively recent. It stems from the power and influence of academic departments and the growth of scientific medicine.

Relatively few people enter medical school with the idea that they should make a contribution to the sum of human knowledge; few aspire to win a Nobel prize. Yet all aspirants to consultant posts and particularly those who wish to teach are expected to be able to point to a number of publications. All young men and women who seek advancement in medicine must be able to produce evidence of completed research.

The main thrust of medical research has been into the function of the body, particularly as it is illuminated by disorder, and into the mechanisms and therapy of disease. Epidemiology – population health – is concerned with origins rather than with mechanisms. It has made and will continue to make greater contributions to the health of communities, as distinct from individuals, than curative medicine.

Research is broadly of two sorts, observational and experimental. Observational research relies on the careful collection of data and its interpretation. It maps the association of events and can generate hypotheses regarding cause. It is generally necessary to test these hypotheses by experiment in which the effects of single factors can be isolated for study.

There has been a considerable growth in operational research in health services which is partly a response to economic pressures. Such research is largely observational and its usefulness is, at the moment, diminished by the lack of tools to measure cost-benefit. While costs are easily computed, benefits can often only be assessed by judgements as to the value or quality of life.

Despite a growing volume of valuable research, the sociology of health, of medicine and the application of behavioural science to the problems of illness have been relatively neglected. A reorientation of the medical profession towards care and support requires a firm base from which to proceed.

It is, however, neither reasonable nor feasible to expect that all doctors will engage in formal research. Most will, or should, attempt to audit their work, to examine what they do. All should try to keep abreast of the major advances in knowledge and the profession can be proud of the effort and enthusiasm with which they undertake this task.

An important number of doctors must continue to pursue new knowledge. Academic departments and universities have a leading part to play in this. One of the present dangers is that the isolation of medical schools from the university and (this applies particularly to departments of general practice) reduces the likelihood of multi-disciplinary approaches to research.

It is almost impossible to write or talk about medical research without paying lip-service to a multi-disciplinary approach, but nonetheless the advantages of bringing different skills, and even more important different perspectives, to bear upon familiar problems can hardly be overemphasised.

While it has been said that the proper application of our present knowledge could, in the short term, make a greater contribution to health than further research, without research medicine would die. Research offers the possibility of rebirth; without it, senescence and death become inevitable. The survival of medicine depends upon the continuing and continuous pursuit of truth: research must not be confined to those things that appear immediately relevant.

Medical Education

Returning to the thesis that doctors are in conflict with society and are making less than their potential contribution to the well-being of their fellow men and women it is necessary to suggest a remedy.

It is some years since I outgrew the notion that education

is the panacea for the world's ills but it is clearly important as an instrument of change. This importance is, in the short term, more theoretical than practical since not only are universities and medical schools, like all great institutions, resistant to change but the effects of change cannot become felt for at least a generation.

Somerville and Ross, in one of their books, refer to trying to load an unwilling red setter into the well of a jaunting car, as attempting to lift a mixture of jelly and lead. Those who try to change institutions, even to institute modest curriculum change, do not find that their shining lances puncture pretentious balloons: they find them blunted and ineffective against a large mass of jelly and lead.

This gloom is not entirely justified. As a profession, doctors take education seriously. There is a flourishing Association for the Study of Medical Education, academic departments are emerging and in every school, even in the most conservative, there is a small body of concerned teachers. More energy has been expended on the setting of educational objectives in faculties of medicine than in any other professional or indeed non-professional school.

There is widespread recognition of the need for change, for reorientation, for different emphases. The problem of translating intent into useful action is, however, more than reallocation of curriculum time to relatively neglected aspects. It depends fundamentally upon a body of teachers which demonstrate, not only on its lips but in its lives, adherence to new values. As Marinker has pointed out, even more important than the stated curriculum is the 'hidden curriculum' – the values which teachers powerfully, continuously and unconsciously transmit to their students.[1]

The danger is, that despite declarations of intent, a hidden curriculum vested in traditional attitudes could effectively prevent any real or significant change. Change depends upon achieving a critical mass of teachers committed to new values who recognise that the effects of their teaching will not become apparent until a large number of their students are practising their profession. This over-simple statement takes no account of the gradualness of change. The changes now taking place in our schools are continuous. Progress is not by means of occasional convulsive heaves, designated as major curriculum reviews, but by a steady and continuing process of adaptation and renewal. There is a lot of evidence that this process is alive.[2]

There is, throughout the world, intense competition for medical school places. This is no doubt in part due to an aspiration to enjoy the income and position which accompany being a doctor. However, I am sure that for many, if not most, the possibility of a career which can be seen as useful and as making a contribution to the quality of life of other people is a major attraction. As always, the young are idealistic, and being a surgeon is much more attractive than manufacturing or selling electrical appliances. Despite forecasts of diminishing job opportunity, more imminent in Ireland than in the United Kingdom, there has been, as yet, no diminution in the number of applicants.

Until fairly recently anyone who wished to study medicine, provided they had had a privileged education and modest academic ability, was likely to be able to do so. This situation has changed because secondary education has become much more widely available and many more children are going on to complete secondary education. Furthermore, university grants make the study of medicine economically possible.

Accompanying this flood of young men and women wishing to study medicine has been a growing criticism of present methods of selection. Some of this represents dissatisfaction with the end product and the profession.

In the UK an almost universal requirement is high grades in scientific subjects in state examinations. Effectively this means that the decision to seek a place in medical school is made at the age of fifteen or sixteen and that the remaining two years at school are spent in assiduous study of a narrow spectrum of scientific disciplines. The humanities are neglected and success is measured by GCE A-level grades obtained. It can be argued without much difficulty that this process tends to produce convergent thinkers, skilled in the assimilation and regurgitation of knowledge: by corollary, it is assumed that it discriminates against divergent thinkers and stifles originality and critical thought. There is little evidence that the corollary is true but it is certain that an interest in the humanities, in art and in literature can only be pursued as a spare time activity.

Some medical schools still interview. There is no evidence that this improves selection and a strong, perhaps unjustified feeling, that it favours short hair, doctor's children, the middle classes and the articulate. A study of the available literature would suggest that while the present method may in many respects be unsatisfactory, no validated alternative is, at present, available.[3] As somebody with a responsibility for admissions, I would say that the present system has the great strength of being, in a sense, demonstrably fair. It might be fairer to set minimum qualifications and then to draw lots — a method that has been used in Holland.

Because selection is largely based upon A-levels, it favours schools which pride themselves on academic success and pupils who are prepared to specialise early and to study hard. For many adolescents getting into medical school, rather than becoming a doctor, has become the goal.

The majority of medical students go straight from school to university. Those who decide relatively late in life, which may be no older than seventeen or eighteen, that they wish to read medicine, can only do so by further study to produce the necessary A-levels or a first class science degree. If their original background was the humanities, they are at a considerable disadvantage. It is worth remarking that some of our most distinguished clinical scientists came into medicine from the classics. While some medical schools favour mature students, many take the view that such people have already made a career choice, and in the case of those over thirty, that training them as doctors is bad economics.

It is certain that those who enter our medical schools are intelligent. Academic failure during the course is rare and those who do not end up as doctors have usually opted out because of uncertainty about career choice, disillusion or occasionally because of illness.

Women in Medicine

Between 30 and 40 per cent of present-day medical students are women, and the proportion is tending to increase. Women have a particular, valuable and unique contribution to make which has not been generally recognised.

As is not surprising, in a profession which is authoritarian, paternalistic and has more recently acquired, or believes it has, a scientific basis, women have been and are, seriously disadvantaged. Despite their considerable numbers they are poorly represented in surgery, as specialist physicians, as heads of academic departments in medical schools, as deans and as presidents of Royal Colleges. Their intelligence is at least as great, their application often greater than that of their male contemporaries.

The hidden discrimination stems, at least in part, from cultural conceptions which, unable to see the witch doctor or the priest as female, have unwittingly endorsed and strengthened the hand of a male-dominated profession.

The problems facing those who wish to combine a career with raising a family are largely ignored. Higher training schemes (including vocational training for general practice), which lead to qualification as somebody fit and entitled to accept unsupervised responsibility, are mostly whole time. They are normally undertaken between the ages of twenty-five and thirty-five, when most women will wish to begin their families and during which children will be small and dependent. As a result, few women have successfully brought up their children and been able to train for consultant posts.

Medicine is the poorer. In her relationship with patients a woman cannot easily be invested with paternalistic authority. The transaction between doctor and patient is immediately more equal. In addition, largely as a result of our cultural mores, women are not, and certainly are seen as much less, interested in personal advancement and financial gain.

Women clearly have special advantages and special concern in caring for other women and for children, and in these specialties, particularly paediatrics, are relatively well represented. They are more practical, less easily shocked: their feet are more firmly on the ground and they are less easily distracted by theoretical considerations of doubtful relevance. Whether these differences are determined by gender, genes or our environment is immaterial. Women are needed in medicine.

The Goals of Medical Education

The nature of our doctors is determined by the characteristics of those who enter training and the education which they subsequently receive. The failings of doctors have been blamed upon faulty selection and wrongheaded education. Good selection and proper training imply that those responsible have a clear idea of the desired end result. Little of the criticism has stemmed from a clear concept of what the end product should be. This is in part a result of the inherent difficulty of defining the nature of a doctor, who may be not only general practitioner or surgeon, but biochemist or medical administrator. This, in turn, has led to the notion of undergraduate education being confined to the production of a basic doctor, who requires further training, rather than to the qualification of a safe general practitioner.

Everyone would agree that a doctor should possess appropriate knowledge. By comparison with skills, and even more by comparison with attitudes, appropriate knowledge can be defined, described and assessed. Because it can be defined and assessed it is overvalued: students know that they fail their examinations for want of knowledge. Unfortunately, knowledge is evanescent unless reinforced by daily use. Furthermore, appropriate knowledge in medicine is continually changing. Examinations ensure that candidates possess knowledge at the time of the examination but do not guarantee that candidates will retain and refurbish their knowledge or that they will be motivated to continue to learn. In the long term the quality of a doctor will be determined not by his knowledge at any particular time but by his behaviour, his motivation to care, to keep up to date, to continue to learn. Medical educators can only inculcate commitment by example. If the profession has changed its character the reasons may be sought in alterations in the nature of the inputs, the raw material, those entering medical schools. Their background, their aspirations and the value of the society from which they spring may be different from those of previous generations. Nevertheless we know that medical education produces doctors stamped in the image of their teachers and medical schools are major determinants of the values of young doctors.

This book is about outcomes: it is an attempt to examine the role of the doctor. Unless this is understood, clarified and agreed, medical education will continue to concentrate on its process and as a result produce doctors ill fitted for their future as servants of our society.

17 FATHER FIGURE OR PLUMBER

Methods of Payment

As a whole doctors are very reluctant to accept that the way in which they are paid influences what they do. Nonetheless they fight energetically to retain the status quo. The Irish Medical Association, when in negotiation with government, seeking that practitioners should be paid on an item-for-service basis, invited articulate opponents of salaried services to address the Association. These doctors had the advantage of speaking to the converted and by the judicious use of terms such as socialised medicine and state control, guaranteed an enthusiastic response. Equally, there are doctors in the National Health Service who regard fee as a dirty word and would be deeply offended if it were suggested that the payment of fees would alter their behaviour.

Those who are paid by means of salary are motivated to reduce their work to the minimum consistent with avoiding dismissal and, if appropriate, ensuring promotion. This tendency may be effectively counteracted by the need for approbation by seniors, the need to earn the gratitude of others or by the need to live with a self which sets high standards and may be obsessional in regard to work. For these reasons payment by salary does not inevitably lead to minimal work but the lack of financial incentive is nonetheless important.

Payment by salary encourages delegation. Delegation has become a feature of practice in the NHS. Out of hours work is delegated to deputising services, dressings and injections are delegated to the nurse, education of mothers to health visitors, deliveries to midwives, problems to social workers, operations to juniors. This has been granted respectability under the guise of the development of a team approach. No one would wish to argue that the intelligent use of the varying talents and experience of different individuals is undesirable. It not only makes the best use of available skills, but also creates opportunities for learning and ultimately provides a better service. It is however dangerous to ignore the reasons, other than better care, which may underlie the act of delegation. Delegation or referral may represent recognition of a need which is better met by somebody else, a recognition of one's own limitations; but it may represent either idleness or rejection. In the case of those who are paid by salary, the less they do the better off they are in terms of both money and leisure. There is little incentive to pay routine visits to the elderly. There is a positive gain in encouraging patients to come to the surgery, and the number of home visits in relation to surgery attendances has steadily fallen and continues to do so. Doctors exert considerable pressure on their patients – pressure which is sometimes resented – to come to the surgery, or to bring feverish children to the health centre, rather than to request a visit.

In Ireland, where general practitioners are paid by fee, similar pressures are generally less and home visits form a much larger proportion of doctors' work. To ascribe this solely to the effect of different methods of payment would, however, ignore other differences which may be equally or even more important. Traditional perceptions and expectations of patients may not be identical, although probably similar; scattered populations with poor public transport may use doctors in a different way; there is a relative dearth in Ireland of other professionals to support doctors.[1] In the United States, where doctors are predominantly paid by fees, it may be virtually impossible to find a doctor who will make a house call because they erode so much time. Americans visiting in the United Kingdom or coming to live here are usually both amazed and delighted to find doctors willing to come to the house. Many American doctors work extremely long hours, driven, it sometimes seems, by an almost insatiable appetite for money which is the mark of success. Their critics have drawn attention to the extent to which doctors themselves determine their workload and the extent to which this may not be fully justified by clinical indications.

Doctors who are paid by fee are discouraged from delegating because such delegation diminishes their income. As a result they may be encouraged to undertake responsibilities for which they have been inadequately trained. In addition delegation has sometimes been perceived as diminishing the patient's view of the doctor's competence. This is particularly true in the United States, where in the absence of general practice, the patient selects an appropriate specialist. Such specialists deal with undifferentiated problems; in a sense they are general practitioners working in a restricted field. As a result they may not acquire expertise in the rare, the really difficult, the unusual. A paediatrician in America will see three times as many children as his practitioner colleague in the UK, but most of the children will have common and not very serious problems. The specialist paediatrician in the UK sees, by referral, the difficult problems of as many as fifty or even a hundred general practitioners and his experience of the relatively uncommon and the difficult is that much greater. An unhappy result of undertaking responsibilities for which practitioners lack experience or training is unnecessary morbidity and mortality. The American enthusiasm for recertification of doctors and the emergence of the Professional Standards Review Organisation (PSRO) is partly a response to the variation in the standard of hospital care, which is much greater than in the United Kingdom.

While payment by salary provides a disincentive to work – the less you do, the better off you are – payment by fee provides an incentive to create work. Governments who pay doctors by fee are haunted by the possibility of abuse: looking across the Atlantic at the Medicaid and Medicare programmes, their fears would appear to be justified. It is very difficult to control the creation of work because, not only may returns be falsified, but there is an almost insatiable demand for services. It may be permissible to accept a mother's statement on the telephone that her second child now has measles, to provide simple advice and reassurance and to offer to see the child should she become concerned. Equally it may be proper to see the child daily in order to provide adequate reassurance and comfort, to examine the ears and chest to exclude complications. In a fee-paying society, if the fees are not a deterrent or are paid by the state, such behaviour may be perceived as being attentive. 'Such a nice young doctor, so attentive!' There are natural checks and balances and those who pay their doctor soon get wise to doctors who over-visit. On the other hand, the state is obliged to rely on deviance from the norm and doctors whose visiting or consultation rates are markedly in excess of those of their peers must expect to be called to account for the difference.

The effects of fees on behaviour are subtle and while familiar to those who have worked in different systems and to those who have been to both Harley Street and hospital outpatients clinics, have been neglected as a subject for research. Doctors generally tend to deny that they have any major effect and provide alternative, and sometimes valid, explanations for differences between systems of care. A doctor who is interested in his work, competent and caring, is likely to provide a good service regardless of how much or in what way he is paid. Habits which are learnt early are persistent and it is at least arguable that the disappearance of competition for patients and the diminished need to court their approval has altered the behaviour of doctors. The generation of doctors which staffed the infant health service and brought to it the values and habits of a different era is now retiring and this may be the reason that a change which has been gradual seems to have been relatively abrupt.

No perfect way of paying doctors exists, but a good system must provide reasonable security as reward for normal work and add modest incentives for additional duties. Money can be used selectively to encourage behaviours. The introduction of a standard obstetric record card in Ireland improved antenatal care because the completed card is the method of obtaining payment. Money is deducted if less than a minimum number of attendances is recorded or if essential data, such as the blood group, is omitted. In the United Kingdom the general practitioner 'charter' of 1966 recognised that payment could be used creatively and introduced fees for night calls. Unfortunately these fees have often been used to finance deputising services and have not generally motivated doctors to provide their own 'on-call' service. Nonetheless suitable incentives can be used to modify the behaviour of doctors as well as the behaviour of children and of plumbers.

Doctors' Income

Doctors' incomes in the United Kingdom have recently and dramatically declined in both absolute and relative terms. The reduction has not been evenly spread: whole time hospital specialists have suffered the most, and non-consultant hospital doctors the least. Indeed the financial position of junior doctors has been transformed for the better in my professional lifetime.

It is a legitimate expectation of those who belong to a learned profession that they should, as a reward for the academic application which has selected them for training and because of the length of their apprenticeship, be paid more than most others in our society. A case for high income can also be made on the grounds of great responsibility. Doctors do, from time to time, carry responsibility for other people's lives.

The idealist may argue that the privilege of being allowed to earn a livelihood in such an interesting way should be reward enough. There is little doubt that under a totalitarian regime most doctors, offered the choice between working on the factory floor or continuing to practise their profession, would, regardless of the fact that their income would be the same whichever they chose, opt to continue as doctors. Nonetheless paying doctors nothing or little more than manual workers enhances the risk that they will conceive of their role as confined to human plumbing, and ensure that they will seek overtime payments, and from time to time withdraw their labour.

If our society expects from its doctors a high standard of service in the best tradition of medicine as a learned profession, it must recognise and encourage such exceptional behaviour by exceptional rewards. At the moment the diminution in doctors' earnings has encouraged non-professional behaviour which in its turn has diminished the chance of higher pay. This is a spiral which unless checked must inevitably lead to the destruction of medicine as a learned profession and to a reduction in the quality of our health services.

A solution must rest on action by both sides. For their part, doctors cannot afford to further diminish their position and to draw still more upon the credit they have inherited. There is a fund of good will, of gratitude, of respect, which although still large, is exhaustible. Every threat of strike action, every unseemly confrontation, diminishes its stock. Doctors must be seen to recognise that their special position is conditional on special behaviour.

For its part society must be prepared to recognise that it is both unreasonable and against its best interests to expect from doctors dedicated and unstinting service without adequate payment. The crisis in doctors' pay is recent. It is partly due to present levels of taxation and the major movement towards an egalitarian society. The demands of doctors in the United Kingdom are not unreasonable. The demands of doctors elsewhere are a measure of their insecurity rather than their poverty.

Professional Service

The rejection of paternalism explicit in 'I don't want a father figure' is an indictment of the unjustified assumption of authority. Acceptable authority must be justified by virtue of superior status, knowledge or learning, or be granted as a consequence of a democratic process of choice. A profession whose claims to be learned are seen to be dubious, whose status is diminishing and whose members behave without proper sanction in an authoritarian way (sometimes in an inverse relationship to their knowledge and skills – those with least knowledge being the most dogmatic), must anticipate rejection.

Science without caring is inhuman, care without science is dangerous. Is it too late to restore a profession whose motto is 'Cum scientia caritas'?

Most of us from time to time have met, or been cared for by doctors, who despite their imperfections, came close to the ideal. Ideal doctors are competent; they know their job and usually provide evidence that this is so. They are also characterised by transparent concern and their commitment to individuals and their problems is, at least for the duration of the consultation, total and complete: they mind.

Is it possible to ensure that doctors are both caring and competent? Is it reasonable, or feasible, to demand from doctors a different code of behaviour; a commitment to the needs of their fellow men and women which is of a different order from that of most people? It would certainly be wrong to assume that commitment of this sort is, could or should, be exclusive to doctors. Many ordinary people, especially those who choose to work with the underprivileged, demonstrate every day that compassion is still alive in our society. Many professionals, especially nurses and social workers, much less well paid than doctors, shame doctors by their concern.

To settle for doctors as plumbers would imply that a good service could be ensured by adequate training certified by examination and disciplined by regulation, recertification and the threat of litigation. Such an approach conjures up visions of Huxley's *Brave New World*, or Orwell's *Nineteen Eighty-Four*.

On the other hand if doctors are to provide a service different in kind from that supplied by fishmongers, mechanics or plumbers, they must be motivated to do so. Genes may have some part in determining the sort of people we are, but in general, behaviour is a product of the influence of the groups in which we live. Honesty is determined more by our upbringing and our own subsequent view of ourselves as honest than the risks of imprisonment. A doctor is unlikely to provide a compassionate, caring service unless he believes himself to be a compassionate person.

One of the disadvantages of egalitarian societies is that the erosion of privilege may also erode the notion of service as the justification for a special position. Lacking a dogma, either Christian or Marxist, which provides a point of reference, it is difficult to demand anything other than behaviours which accord with the lowest common denominator of a particular society. Doctors are part of society and the values which medical students bring to medicine are those of their families, their social class and their schools. If these values are to change, our society will have to change. Such change is by no means impossible: it is characteristic of growing old that there always seems to have been considerable change, invariably for the worse, in any particular lifetime. From the vantage point of middle age, there seem to have been many changes in my lifetime which have been, and are, good. Nonetheless, I fear that there are in our society fewer doctors who believe that service is the price of privilege.

Richard Titmuss had this to say:

> I regard the National Health Service Act as one of the most unsordid and civilised actions in the history of health and welfare policy. It put family doctors on a footing with university teachers, and patients on a footing with university students. Both professional groups – of doctors and teachers – are expected to give generously of what they know without a price being put on time or knowledge. The presumption in the relationship is thus more social than economic. Moreover, both are expected to give more than they can conceivably give because knowledge advances, men are not computers, and there are only twenty-four hours in the day. In this sense, professional service is never stationary, it knows no limits and there is no resting place or terminus . . .[2]

In advocating that doctors should recognise that service is the price of privilege and that medicine requires 'caritas', not only as a condition of survival as a learned profession, but in order to provide proper care, I lay myself open to the charge of naïve idealism. Such aspirations are not only unrealistic but ludicrous.

While it is indeed ludicrous to expect of doctors a form of sainthood, society will settle for much less. It does not expect perfection from its doctors. If they demonstrate their concern for the individual they will be excused many of their shortcomings. Their liability to be held to account for failure is limited.

Envoi

Sir George Pickering, who has referred to medicine as being at a crossroads, fears that the profession has already chosen the downhill road which will ultimately reduce a learned profession to a technological trade union.[3] He fears that doctors will be reduced to human plumbers. Those who seek to demystify medicine, who resent the unjustified assumption of authority and doctors' special position may welcome and encourage such a trend.

There is a course which the profession can follow which lies between human plumbing and paternalism. It is possible to combine technical competence with knowledge of its limitations: possible to recognise human needs and to allow to Everyman his autonomy and his right to human dignity.

The doctor can still aspire as his forefathers did to mediate between the patient and his illness. He can enhance the prospects of cure, diminish unreasonable fear and assist in the process of adaptation. This demands more than knowledge of disease; it demands concern and awareness of people as individual, unique, human beings. It requires both wisdom and judgement, virtues seldom praised in the seventies.

Neither father figures nor plumbers, it is possible that doctors may again earn the respect of the society they serve.

REFERENCES

1 The Role of the Doctor

1. George Pickering, 'Medicine at the Crossroads: Learned Profession or Technological Trades Union?', *Proceedings of the Royal Society of Medicine*, 70 (1977), 16-20.

2. J.P. Kevany *et al.*, 'Goals for Medical Education — The Community Viewpoint', *Journal of the Irish Medical Association* (1977), 70, 380.

3. Julian Tudor Hart, *Practice. A Handbook of Primary Medical Care*, London, Kluwer-Harrap Handbooks, 1977, 4.5-04.

2 The Nature of Health

1. M. Stacey, Health and Health Policy, Social Science Research Council, 1977.

2. Ivan Illich, *Medical Nemesis. The Expropriation of Health,* London, Calder and Boyars, 1974; Rene Dubos, *The Mirage of Health*, London, Allen & Unwin, 1960.

3. Talcott Parsons, *The Social System*, London, Routledge & Kegan Paul, 1951.

3 The Doctor and the Patient

1. Thomas McKeown, *The Role of Medicine: Dream, Mirage or Nemesis?,* The Rock Carling Fellowship, London, Nuffield Provincial Hospital Trust, 1976.

2. R. Klein, *Complaints against Doctors. A Study in Professional Accountability*, London, Charles Knight, 1973.

3. K.J. Mann, 'The Role of the Family and Community Health Centre', *Bulletin of the New York Academy of Medicine,* 42 (1966), no. 2, 742.

4. J.S. McCormick, 'Motives in Medicine', *Proceedings of the Royal Society of Medicine,* 68 (1974).

5. Kenneth Edwards, 'Personal View', *British Medical*

Journal, 2 (1976), no. 6041, 938.
6. G.K. Hodgkin, 'Behaviour – the Community and the General Practitioner', *Journal of the Royal College of General Practitioners,* 19 (1970), 5-11.
7. J.L.W. Price, 'The Patient's Morale', *Lancet,* 1 (1977) 533.
8. Working Party of the Royal College of General Practitioners, *The Future of the General Practitioner; Learning and Teaching,* 1972.
9. G.V. Stimson, in Margaret Stacey (ed.), *Sociology of the NHS,* University of Keele, 1976.
10. A. Davis and G. Horobin (eds.), *Medical Encounters,* London, Croom Helm, 1976.
11. A. Cartwright, *Social Class Variations in Health Care and in the Nature of General Practitioner Consultations,* London, Institute for Social Studies Health Care, 1975.
12. E. Blake Moore, 'Anaesthesia and Analgesia – Current Researches', *Lancet,* 55 (1976), no. 5, 756.
13. J.C. Hoffman, *Lancet,* I (1977) 801.

4 Diagnosis

1. D.C. Morell and C.J. Wale, *Journal of the Royal College of General Practitioners,* 26 (1976), 398-403.
2. R.H.V. Jones, *Journal of the Royal College of General Practitioners,* 26, (1976), 410.
3. Ann Cartwright, *Patients and Their Doctors – A Study of General Practice,* London, Routledge & Kegan Paul, 1967.
4. I.R. McWhinney, 'Problem Solving and Decision Making in Primary Medical Care' (Albert Wander Lecture), *Proceedings of the Royal Society of Medicine,* 65 (1972), 934-8.
5. P.S. Byrne and B.E.L. Long, *Doctors Talking to Patients,* London, HMSO, 1976.
6. Royal College of General Practitioners, Research Committee Study, *Journal of the Royal College of General Practitioners,* I (1958), 107-28.
7. I.S.L. Loudon, in 'Trends in General Practice', *British Medical Journal,* London (1977).
8. 'Reducing Doctors' Errors', *British Medical Journal,* I (1977), 1178.

9. M.F. Moore, J.H. Barber, E.T. Robinson and T.R. Taylor, *Lancet,* I (1973), 817-19; W.O. Spitzer, D.L. Sackett, J.C. Sibley, R.S. Roberts, M. Gent, D.J. Kergin, B.C. Hacklett and A. Olynich, *New England Journal of Medicine,* 290 (1974), 251-56.

5 Treatment

1. 'Life Cycle of an FPIO', *British Medical Journal,* I (1977), 670.
2. W.V. Slack, *Lancet,* II (1977), 240.
3. K.C. Easton, *Proceedings of the Royal Society of Medicine,* 63 (1970), 1321.

6 Reassurance

1. A. Cartwright, *Patients and their Doctors,* London, Routledge & Kegan Paul, 1967.
2. P.S. Byrne, and B.E.L. Long, *Doctors Talking to Patients,* London, HMSO, 1976.

7 Problems of Living

1. G.W. Brown, M.N. Ni Brolchain, and T. Harris, 'Social Class and Psychiatric Disturbance among Women in an Urban Population', *Sociology,* 9 (1975), 225-54.
2. N. Kessel, *British Medical Journal,* 2 (1965), 1265.
3. Eric Wilkes, in *Practice – A Handbook of Primary Medical Care,* London,Kluwer-Harrap Handbooks.
4. A.M.W. Ward, 'Mortality and Bereavement', *British Medical Journal,* I (1976), 700.
5. The Medical Sociology Research Centre, University College, Swansea, 'Prescribing in General Practice', Royal College of General Practitioners, Supp. 1, 26 (1976).
6. M. Balint, *The Doctor, His Patient and the Illness,* 2nd edn., London, Pitman Medical, 1964.

8 Counselling

1. P.S. Byrne and B.E.L. Long, *Doctors Talking to Patients,* London, HMSO, 1976.
2. Andrew Malleson, *Need Your Doctor Be So Useless,* London, Allen & Unwin, 1973.

9 Sickness

1. Talcott Parsons, *The Social System*, Glencoe, Illinois, Routledge & Kegan Paul, 1951.
2. Sir George Pickering, *Creative Malady*, Allen & Unwin, London, 1974.

10 Prevention

1. Thomas McKeown and C.R. Lowe, *Introduction to Social Medicine*, London, Blackwell Science, 1974.
2. J.M.G. Wilson and F. Jungner, 'Principles and Practice of Screening for Disease', Public Health Papers No. 34, WHO Geneva (1968).
3. L.M. Irwig, *Lancet*, II (1974), 1307.
4. Report of a Joint Working Party of the Royal College of Physicians of London and the British Cardiac Society 'Prevention of Coronary Heart Disease', *Journal of the Royal College of Physicians*, 10 (1976), no. 3.
5. R. Doll and R. Peto, 'Mortality among Doctors in Different Occupations', *British Medical Journal*, I (1977), 1433.
6. P. Puska, 'World Health',Oct. 12 WHO, Geneva (1976).
7. Aengus O'Rourke and Keith Wilson-Davis, 'Smoking and School Children', *Journal of the Royal College of General Practitioners*, 20 (1970), no. 101, 354-60.

11 Care

1. J. Egbert, G.E. Battit, C.E. Welch and M.K. Bartlett, *New England Journal of Medicine*, 270 (1964), 825.

12 Old Age

1. L.J. Opit and S.M. Shaw, *Lancet*, 2 (1976), 1127.
2. Royal College of Physicians Working Party 'Care of the Elderly', a Report of the Standing Committee of Members of the Royal College of Physicians, *Journal of the Royal College of Physicians*, 10, no. 3 (April 1976).

13 Psychiatry and Obstetrics

1. *Report on the Work of the Prison Department 1976* (1977), Cmnd 6877, London, HMSO, 1977.

2. Margaret Wynn and Arthur Wynn, *Prevention of Handicap of Perinatal Origin: An Introduction to French Policy,* Foundation for Education and Research in Child Bearing, London, 1976.

3. P.M. Dunn, *Lancet,* I (1976), 790.

4. C.H. Kempe, Armstrong Lecture, University of Colorado Medical Center, 1975.

5. S. Bourne, *Journal of the Royal College of General Practitioners,* 16 (1968), 103.

14 General Practice

1. R.M.S. McConaghey, *Journal of The Royal College of General Practitioners,* 22 (1972), 775-88.

2. F. Honigsbaum, *Journal of The Royal College of General Practitioners,* 22 (1972), 429-51.

3. *The General Practitioner in Ireland,* Report of the Consultative Council on General Medical Practice, Government Publications Office, Dublin, 1973.

4. T.F. Fox, *Lancet,* I (1960), 743-60.

5. Julian Tudor Hart, 'The Inverse Care Law', *Lancet,* I (1971) 405-12.

15 The Doctor and Society

1. *Report of the Royal Commission on Medical Education,* (Todd Report), Cmnd. 3569, London, HMSO 1968.

2. *Committee on Child Health Services, Fit for the Future,* London, HMSO, 1976.

3. J. Freeman and P.S. Byrne, *Assessment of Postgraduate Training in General Practice,* Society for Research into Higher Education, 1973.

16 Research and Education

1. M. Marinker, 'Medical Education and Human Values', *Journal of the Royal College of General Practitioners,* 24 (1974), 445.

2. *Basic Medical Education in the British Isles,* Nuffield Provincial Hospitals Trust, London, 1977.

3. *The Selection of Medical Students,* WHO Copenhagen, 1971.

17 Father Figure or Plumber

1. J.S. McCormick and S.A. Allwright, 'A Comparison of General Practice in Britain and Ireland', *Journal of the Royal College of General Practitioners,* 27 (1977), 271-4.

2. R.M. Titmuss, 'Role of the Family Doctor Today in the Context of Britain's Social Services', *Lancet,* I (1965), 1.

3. Sir George Pickering, 'Medicine at the Crossroads: Learned Profession or Technological Trades Union?' *Proceedings of the Royal Society of Medicine,* 70 (1977), 16-20.

INDEX